MENTAL DISEASES

AND

THEIR MODERN TREATMENT

BY

SELDEN HAINES TALCOTT, A.M., M.D., Ph.D.

Medical Superintendent of the Middletown State Homeopathic Hospital in Middletown, N. Y.; Professor of Mental Diseases in the New York Homeopathic Medical College and Hospital

---

INDIAN EDITION

B. Jain Publishers (P) Ltd.
USA—EUROPE—INDIA

MENTAL DISEASES AND THEIR MODERN TREATMENT

9th Impression: 2013

> **NOTE FROM THE PUBLISHERS**
> Any information given in this book is not intended to be taken as a replacement for medical advice. Any person with a condition requiring medical attention should consult a qualified practitioner or therapist.

All rights reserved. No part of this book may be reproduced, stored in a retrieval system or transmitted, in any form or by any means, mechanical, photocopying, recording or otherwise, without any prior written permission of the publisher.

© with the Publisher

Published by Kuldeep Jain for
B. JAIN PUBLISHERS (P) LTD.
1921/10, Chuna Mandi, Paharganj, New Delhi 110 055 (INDIA)
Tel.: +91-11-4567 1000 • *Fax:* +91-11-4567 1010
Email: info@bjain.com • *Website:* **www.bjain.com**

Printed in India by
J.J. Offset Printers

ISBN: 978-81-319-0825-9

I DEDICATE THIS WORK TO THE

CLASS OF 1900

OF THE

NEW YORK HOMEOPATHIC MEDICAL COLLEGE

AND HOSPITAL

AND

TO ALL OTHER EARNEST STUDENTS OF

MENTAL MEDICINE

PREFACE

During the past twenty-five years I have been engaged in the practical work of ministering to the needs of the insane. This work has resulted in a gradual development of that form of treatment which has been designated as "The Hospital Idea". In other words, the asylum has given place to the hospital in the protection and restoration of mental invalids. The fact is now generally recognized that the insane man is a sick man, and needs for his comfort and cure the application of such means as are ordinarily used for the benefit of the sick in a modern general hospital. Acting under this belief, our patients have been favored with such treatment as may be best exemplified by skilled physicians, trained nurses, and hospital methods and appliances. At the Middletown State Homeopathic Hospital there have been afforded not only hospital measures for the recuperation of the mentally sick, but the indicated homeopathic remedy has been applied with conscientious fidelity in each case. Individualization, and hospitalization, and homeopathic treatment, have been the methods pursued in the institutions under my charge during the past quarter of a century. This work embodies, in a series of lectures, a long experience in working for the good of the insane. In it I have tried to explain the nature of the disease under consideration; also its causes, its tendencies, and its conclusions under favorable treatment.

This work is not an exhaustive treatise upon insanity. It consists simply of a few "blaze marks" guiding the way through the wilderness of mental disorder, and into the sunny fields of health. If it shall become an aid to the medical student in the acquisition of knowledge, and to the busy practitioner in the care and cure of the sick, then its purpose will have been accomplished.

THE AUTHOR

Middletown, N. Y., April 1901

PREFACE TO FIRST INDIAN EDITION

This book embodies, in a series of lectures, a long experience in working for the good of those who suffer from mental derangement. The reprint of the book is undertaken in the hope that it shall become an aid to the students and practitioners of Homeopathy in the care and cure of the insane. The publishers offer it to the profession and trust that this purpose will be served.

PUBLISHERS

CONTENTS

LECTURE I

THE HUMAN BRAIN

Its coverings, divisions and subdivisions, weight, functions, localization of functions, operations, uses, abuses, and capabilities   1–20

LECTURE II

THE INSANE DIATHESIS OR ABNORMAL TENDENCIES OF THE HUMAN MIND

Definition. Causes, inherited and acquired. Evidences, avoidance, and treatment 21–40

LECTURE III

SLEEP, SLEEPLESSNESS AND THE CURE OF INSOMNIA

What is sleep? The Condition for sleep. The natural causes of sleep. Causes of insomnia. Suggestions for the induction of sleep. Remedies 41–57

LECTURE IV

HISTORY AND CLASSIFICATION OF INSANITY, THEORIES, DEFINITIONS, AND REQUIREMENTS FOR COMMITMENT

History. Classification of insanity. British Classification. American Classification. Theories, Definitions. Requirements for commitment. Contra-indications of commitment 58–80

LECTURE V

MELANCHOLIA

Definition. Causes. Forms. Symptoms, courses and cases. Delusions. Prevalence and prevention. Pathological states . . . 81–110

LECTURE VI

MANIA

Characteristics. Causes. Forms. Symptoms, courses and cases. Pathological states 111–139

CONTENTS

LECTURE VII

DEMENTIA

Nature. Forms. Causes. Symptoms and treatment of acute dementia. Chronic dementia. Masturbatic dementia. Syphilitic dementia. Epileptic dementia. Organic dementia. Alcoholic dementia. Senile dementia. Pathological states 140–160

LECTURE VIII

GENERAL PARESIS

History. Synonyms. Stages, Cases. Causes. Pathology. Diagnosis, prognosis and treatment. Prevention 161–187

LECTURE IX

TREATMENT

At home. In sanitariums or State hospitals. Means for treating the insane, kindness and gentle discipline, rest in bed, enforced protection, exercise, amusement and occupation, artificial feeding, dietetics, moral hygiene, operations, the hospital idea 188–207

LECTURE X

MEDICAL TREATMENT

How to prescribe. Principal remedies for the treatment of melancholia, mania, dementia, and general paresis 208–220

HOSPITAL CONSTRUCTION

Site. Construction of buildings. Solariums. Ventilation, heating and lighting. Protection against fire. Furnishings and decorations. Congregate and ward dining-rooms. Kitchen and bakery building. Boiler house, dynamo plant and laundry. Cold storage building. Outbuildings for stock of various kinds 220–236

COMPENDIUM OF MATERIA MEDICA

Comprising the leading remedies and their principal indications in the treatment of mental disorders 237–310

INDEX OF REMEDIES

WITH THEIR PRINCIPAL SYMPTOMS 311–312

Lecture I

THE HUMAN BRAIN

Three thousand years ago, more or less, there were inscribed above the portals of the temple of Apollo at Delphi these immortal words, "Gnothi Seauton" (γνωθι σεαυτον), which being translated from the original Greek into the present vernacular of the United States, means "Know Thyself". That we may know ourselves better than before, let us consider today the human brain, its functions, its uses, its abuses, and its capabilities.

No one can presume to unfold in all their fullness and perfection the mysterious workings and the marvellous mechanism of the human brain. So intricate a subject can never be fully understood except by the Infinite Mind that planned and brought into action this rarest product of all creation. Still, possibly, we may comprehend in a measure the mechanism of the brain, and by careful study come to understand in some slight degree the uses of that wonderful organ, and also the disastrous effects of its misuse.

We shall proceed to strip off the coverings of the head and pursue our searches to the core, explaining as we pass along, in brief, each part as we find it. This work has, I presume, already been performed by your professor of anatomy, and I shall merely enumerate the component parts of the head in this connection for the sole purpose of drawing your attention to a material structure as an organ of the mind, and then pass to a contemplation of the subtle processes of the mind itself.

The coverings of the brain are three in number:

1. The periostic (above the bone),—namely, the hair, scalp, and muscles.

2. The bony cranium.

3. The sub-osseous,—namely, the membranes lying beneath the skull and over the carebral mass.

The scalp is a thick, tough, tenacious covering, forming the base and ground-work whence springs that luxurious adornment, the human hair. The scalp is thicker than the skin of any other portion of the body. A thick scalp protects the brain from accidental injuries. It is also supposed to prevent a too rapid in-pouring of ideas upon the brain. The scalp is attached to the skull by means of the occipito-frontalis muscle. The latter covers the skull, and has attachments along the crest of the brow, over the eyes, and at the occiput, or back part of the head. It is by means of this muscle that the brows are elevated in token of surprise, or corrugated as an evidence of displeasure or chagrin. The occipito-frontalis muscle is thin even at its extremities or points of insertion. Over the top of the head it is but little more than a thick membrane or flattened tendon.

Beneath the scalp and its controlling muscle, we arrive at the skull, an egg-shaped, bony case, flattened underneath, the forepart of which gives attachments to the face. The skull is composed of flat bones consisting of two layers, an outer and an inner table, and a spongy tissue, known as diploë, between them. Where the walls are very thin there is but a single layer. The vault of the skull presents two minute openings (the parietal foramina) for the passage of small veins. At the base are many openings for the transmission of nerves, and for other purposes. The skull-cap proper is very strong, and built to resist heavy blows. The base of the skull is relatively weak and easily broken. The various bones of the skull are laced or inter-laced together by what are called the sutures in such a way as to oppose the tearing off of any bone by force acting in a single direction.

On removing the skull-cap we arrive at the three sub-osseous coverings called membranes. The first, or that next the skull, is termed the dura mater, which, as compared with the others, is thick and exceedingly tense and firm, resembling in some slight degree a drumhead or piece of parchment. Excepting on the crown, it is closely adherent to the skull, with which it is very intimately associated, as through its outward surfaces the minute vessels which supply the bony casing of the brain with blood find their way. The inner surface of the dura mater, that is, the surface next the brain, is smooth and oily, so to speak, thus relieving the slight friction which takes place between the brain and its protecting citadel, as the former swells into action under the pressure of excitement or subsides into a grateful calm during its appropriate periods for repose. The dura mater forms still another protection for the brain; its density and firmness resisting with vigor all encroachments from without, the splintered fragments of a fractured skull even being held in abeyance in many instances. By these appropriate means the most vital organ of the body is protected from fatal injuries.

The second membrane is termed the arachnoid from its supposed resemblance to a spider's web. It is a single layer of thin, delicate, connective tissue overhanging the convolutions of the brain, and dividing into two the spaces between the organ and the skull. The outer of these is called the subdural space, and the inner the subarachnoid. It was formerly supposed that the arachnoid membrane formed a close sac like the pleura, which envelops the lungs and lines the walls of the thorax, but investigations have tended to disprove this theory. What was supposed to be its outer, or reflected portion, is really one of the layers of the dura mater. The chief uses of the arachnoid seem to be to envelop and in some measure to protect the brain, and to secrete a fluid for the purpose of keeping it in a state best adapted for the proper performance of its functions.

The third membrane, which is discovered as we pursue our explorations, is termed the pia mater, or delicate mother. This, too, like the arachnoid, is a layer of connective tissue, but it performs the work of holding together vast numbers of small arteries and veins that carry on, to a large extent, the circulation of the brain. This membrane is adherent to the brain surfaces, covering closely the convolutions and dipping into the sulci or spaces between them. As the blood vessels pass into the brain from the pia mater like so many little rootlets, the membrane is of course fastened snugly to that organ.

The brain itself is divided into hemispheres. These hemipheres are subdivided into lobes. The hemispheres are separated by the great longitudinal fissure which extends throughout the length of the cerebrum in the middle line, reaching down to the base of the brain in front and behind, but interrupted in the middle by a broad band of white matter termed the corpus callosum. This band unites the hemsipheres like the firm mass which united the Siamese twins.

Each half of the brain is divided into what are called the frontal, parietal, occipital and temporal lobes; and for a fifth lobe we have what is termed the Island of Reil.

After removing the coverings we come to the convolutions. These are separated from each other by depressions called sulci. It is supposed that the deeper the sulci, the greater the brain power. This is not always true, but the deeper the sulci the greater the opportunity for a deposit of gray matter.

Upon the outer surfaces of the convolutions, and on the sides and bottom of the sulci, is a gray matter called the cortical substance. In the gray matter there are five or six layers of nerve cells. Many of these cells are shaped like a pyramid, while some are round and some are elongated. The nerve cells have a nucleus, a plasma, and a surrounding pellicle or skin, and also outreaching tentacles or arms. The entire outfit is called the neuron. Within the cortical substance we find the white fibres which are in reality the connecting wires of communication between the nerve extremities of the body and the neurine batteries of the brain. The nerve fibres convey impressions to the cells, and the cells which receive these impressions act according to the impression which is made.

Besides nerve cells and nerve fibres there is a substance in the brain called the neuroglia. The neuroglia "is a transparent, nucleated, homogeneous, non-fibrillated matrix, somewhat resembling the fibrillated connective tissue of the spinal cord." Supposing you were to put a lot of berries on some strings, and then put them into a glass jar with the ends of the strings hanging over the mouth of the jar, and then fill in the interstices with some syrup, this syrup might represent or typify the neuroglia. After the Almighty had constructed the nerve cells which are the homes and centers of mental activity, and after He had connected them by nerve fibres with the great organs and surfaces of the body, that is, with the external world, He filled up the cracks with neuroglia, which is simply connective tissue, and other supporting material.

Histologically, you will remember that the cerebral mass is composed of gray matter filled with cells of many kinds, of white matter (that is, white nerve lines of communication), and of neuroglia, which is a nucleated mass thrown in for the support of the rest of the brain.

Having plodded through the brain, we arrive at the base,

and, as we expose it to view, we see the longitudinal fissure, the corpus callosum, and its peduncles, the lamina cinerea, the olfactory nerve, the fissure of Sylvius, the anterior perforated space, the optic commissure, the tuber cinereum, the infundibulum, the pituitary body (which is said to be the seat of the soul), the corpora albicantia, the posterior perforated space, and the crura cerebri. Now I trust that you will never forget any of these since I have taken the trouble to bring them to your notice.

From the base of the brain are given off twelve pairs of nerves. These are called nerves of sensation, motion, and special sense, and are the mediums through which impressions, both external and internal, are conveyed to the brain, and through these all orders of the mind to the body are conveyed for execution.

The functions of seeing, smelling, tasting and hearing, are performed by the optic, olfactory, trifacial, and glossopharyngeal nerves. Portions of those just named, and the remainder of the twelve, constitute the nerves of sensation and motion. Some anatomists name but nine pairs of nerves. We prefer a division of twelve, and shall enumerate them as follows:

1. Olfactory,
2. Optic,
3. Motor oculi,
4. Pathetic,
5. Trifacial,
6. Abducens,
7. Facial,
8. Auditory,
9. Glosso-pharyngeal,
10. Pneumogastric,
11. Spinal accessory,
12. Hypoglossal.

There are in the brain five ventricles. The chief of these are the lateral, and those of lesser importance are the third, fourth, and fifth. The lateral are large and occupy a considerable part of the cerebral center, running in a general way lengthwise along the base, but always, according to Hogarth's line of beauty, on a curve. The ventricles are important, because we find in them the choroid plexuses which, when diseased tend to produce sleeplessness, and insanity.

The next in importance to the lateral ventricles is the fourth ventricle. This is bounded in front and below by the medulla, and the reverse of the pons which constitute its floor; above and behind by the cerebellum; in front by the valve of Vieussens, and the superior peduncle; on the side by the restiform bodies, part of the pons, and the lateral lobes of the cerebellum. It is said that diabetes is due to some diseased condition found in the floor of the fourth ventricle.

The third ventricle extends anteriorly along the base of the brain to and between the optic thalami.

The space between the septum lucidum, which is very slight, is called the fifth ventricle.

All the true ventricles communicate with one another; the two lateral with the third, the third with the fourth at the aqueduct of Sylvius, the fourth with the central canal of the spinal cord and with the subarachnoid space.

The significance of the ventricles lies in the fact that effusions occur in them and thus the action of the brain is either impaired, or destroyed.

The cerebellum, or little brain, is supposed to preside over the functions of co-ordination, as they relate to equilibrium, harmony and the symmetrical action of the two parts of the body.

The medulla oblongata is the butt end of the spinal cord. The band of union between this end of the cord, the cerebellum, and the cerebrum is termed the pons varolii.

Viewing the brain from the standpoint of development, we find that it is divided into three parts:

1. The forebrain, consisting of the olfactory lobes, the

cerebral hemispheres, and the parts surrounding the third ventricle.

2. The midbrain, consisting of the corpora quadrigemini, and the crura cerebri.

3. The hindbrain, consisting of the cerebellum, the pons varolii, and the medulla oblongata.

This is the classification of Huxley, and is simple and easily remembered.

The physiological peculiarity of the brain is that it selfishly requires for its proper nourishment about one-sixth of all the blood in the entire body.

The brain in the newborn infant is said to weigh about ten ounces. The average weight of the adult brain ranges from forty to forty-eight ounces. The brain of the celebrated Cuvier weighed over sixty-four ounces, that of Abercrombie sixty-three, while those of Agassiz, Daniel Webster, and a common daylaborer weighed about fifty-three ounces each. The size of any given brain, all other things being equal, determines its power. But the quality must also be considered. This varies greatly. The brain of Gambetta weighed but thirty-six ounces, while the brain of a United States idiot weighed sixty-seven ounces. The difference in the brain power depends not alone upon the size, but also upon the quality. The quality of the brain can generally be determined by its achievements.

Great differences of opinion have existed with regard to the period at which brains attain their full size. Sir William Hamilton asserted that the brain reached its maturity, as to size, at the age of seven years. Other celebrated writers have claimed that the brain matures between the twentieth and thirtieth years. We believe that under ordinary usage the brain matures gradually with the body, and so long as the general system maintains growth, so long the brain may continue to grow. The head of Napoleon was small in youth, but acquired in after life an enormous development. So it seems that the force of an untiring and active brain may assert itself even against its body environments.

We come now to speak of the functions performed by the brain. These may be divided into two classes: (1) Those which preside over and direct the various motions of the body, physical functions, so to speak; (2) the higher or mental functions, wherein are involved cognizance, memory, and judgment.

The action of the brain, in its relation to the body, may be illustrated by comparing it to the action of a spider in relation to its web. This famous animal is usually found at home in the most central portion of its self-constructed domicile. It may be apparently asleep, but if you touch ever so lightly one of the filaments of the spider's web, he instantly takes notice of the fact, and seeks to repair the injuries which have been wrought. So the brain stands like a sleepless Cerberus in the center of the much-diverging nerve fabric, and if you prick a nerve extremity the shock is vibrated with lightning-like rapidity to the brain, and from it goes forth the order to the muscular guardians of the injured part to hold the fort, or to beat a retreat, as may seem best. A good illustration of nerve action is when a boy sits down upon a bent pin, and then gets up again.

Let us now attend to the localization of those functions of the brain which direct and influence the body. By applying the galvanic current to different portions of the exposed brain in the case of a monkey, and carefully noting the effects, it was observed and determined that the excitement of one part of the brain caused movements of the lower limbs of the opposite side, as in walking. By stimulating another portion of the brain, the muscles of the forearm became flexed, while stimulation of another part would cause protrusion of the tongue, etc. Repeated trials enabled the experimenters to mark out on the brain the exact limits of these physical functions, and within the circles thus described, by due stimulus, action in some particular part of the body was invariably excited. Thus were the functions of the brain in their relationships to the functions of the body discovered and localized.

It was also discovered that certain portions of the brain were not used in thus controlling the actions of the body. These unused portions are found in the fore and hind parts of the brain. It is generally believed that in the anterior portion of the brain the intellectual workings are carried on, while in the hind part of the brain are located the centers of the emotions, the passions, and the appetites.

It is an interesting fact that each portion of the brain has its specific and special duty to perform. This fact has been demonstrated by the experiments of Fleurens, Longet, Velpeau, Ferrier, Hitzig, and others. By removing successively portions of the brain in some of the lower animals, the powers of what remained were determined. When the upper lobes of the brain were removed from a pigeon, that bird was deprived of the powers of memory, and will; but it could fly when thrown into the air, it could be roused by a gentle push or pinch, by a light flashed before its eyes, by ammonia held near its nostrils, by a pistol discharged close to its head. By removing another layer of brain tissue the faculty of sight is destroyed, while hearing remains. By removing still another layer the faculty of hearing is destroyed; and again, the power of motion is paralyzed, and so on to the end of the chapter. When we come to excise that center from which the pneumogastric nerve springs, then the heart and lungs are paralyzed and the animal dies.

This is true in all cases except that of the frog. A frog can live for a short time by cutaneous respiration, for scientific purpose, of course. The frog may be decapitated, and all nerve centers removed except those located in the spinal cord, and then if a portion of the belly be irritated with a drop of acid, an attempt will be made by the frog to remove the irritating substance by rubbing it off with his right leg. Now cut off the right leg and you will see an attempt to reach the irritated spot by the stump. Not succeeding, the animal will pause and think it over with his spinal cord, and then you will see him try to remove the acid with his left leg.

We now pass to a consideration of the brain as a seat of mental power,—the temporal kingdom of the mind, the earthly tabernacle of the immortal soul.

Within the convolutions of the brain rest not only the power of guiding and propelling the physical forces, but, also, therein is the seat of a higher power which enables man to control not only his own actions, but to influence and direct the actions of others; to oppose successfully his intellectual vigor and prowess against the crude strength of the lower animals, and against the combative elements of earth and sea and air.

Man's brain, in the first place, takes cognizance of external things through perception or impression. Next he stores away the fruits of cognizance in the wine press and vaults of memory. From these come forth at last the rich essence of judgment, the final result of a subtle and mysterious process. The will executes the mandates of the judgment.

The ancients thought that the brain was but a useless mass of crude matter, a sort of overgrown clam, a mountain snow-cap to keep the rest of the body cool. The modern student finds that the brain, which the ancients despised, has become the chief and most important organ of the human body. The human mind, the occupant of this brain, is the marvel and the mystery of creation. It is swayed by every flitting passion or impression, and yet it is held in steady poise by the calm monitions of reason, of cultivated judgment, and of developed will. In these respects it resembles those wonderous rocking-stones reared by the ancient Druids. You remember that they were so finely balanced that the finger of a child could vibrate them to their centers, and yet they were so firmly poised that the might of an army could not move them from their base. So it is with the human mind which has been thoroughly trained, carefully cultured, and kept by its owner as a pearl without price. The smile of a child can sway it to and fro, while the faggot of martyrdom could not change one jot or tittle of its firm determination.

Let us see how the brain works during the evolution of thought. It is claimed that there are two classes of intellectual faculties,—the knowing, and the reflecting. The knowing faculties are individuality, form, size, weight, coloring, locality etc. The reflecting faculties are comparison, and causality. Each faculty has, it is said, a separate portion of the brain for its home. The memory belongs to each faculty. Hence there are as many kinds of memory as there are homes for the knowing and reflecting faculties. Sometimes by reason of localized brain disease a person may lose the power of recalling a name, or place, or event, and yet may be able to exercise his memory with regard to all the faculties except the one which has been disturbed by disease.

Memory is simply a retentive attribute or power of the mind. The best view to take of memory is to regard it as the holding of a feeling, a thought, or a purpose in the continuous life of the mind. Every thinking act continues, every choice and purpose likewise remain part of the mind's activity. The law of retentiveness in the mind imposes three conditions for a good memory. They are found:

1. In the subject matter of remembrance,
2. In the relationship of each thing remembered to other things in the mind, and,
3. In the care of the mind itself.

The first condition is that the mind accepts readily only what it most needs or wishes to use; therefore, you should get good things to remember. The second is to associate them carefully with things already remembered in such a manner that they may be easily recalled. The third condition, without day-dreaming or mind-wandering, is fixing attention to the subject that you may wish to memorize.

Professor Bain classifies mental activities as follows:

1. The senses—that is, the five senses,
2. The intellect, or the mental processes which are developed between impressions on the one hand and determination on the other,
3. The will, with which the judgment is closely associated.
4. The emotions.

The products of the senses are called sensations. The products of the intellect are ideas, beliefs, imaginings, derived from processes of reasoning and understanding and arriving at the conclusion of judgment. The products of the will are volitions; and the products of the emotions are feelings and passions.

The first step in mental activity is self-consciousness. The mind takes cognizance of an impression produced upon the brain by any of the five senses. When the brain receives an impression from any source, and the mind becomes conscious of it, then there is formed within the mind what are called perceptions. The power of perceiving and comparing is called the intelligence. The intelligence is the mind's faculty of knowing. After receiving various and repeated impressions, and after forming numerous comparison of objects which we often see, we find at last that there has been developed an automatic function, so to speak, and this is known as intuition. Intuition is the faculty of internal perception and internal comprehension. Intuition is a limited sphere of mental phenomena. It is an incomplete knowledge, and thus the faculty of thought is stirred into activity. Thought is the elaborative faculty, the comparative faculty, the faculty of relationships. Well, we put several thoughts together, and let them have a warlike struggle, and this process of fighting, of thoughts rubbing against each other, and concluding either victory or defeat, we call reasoning. After this fight of thoughts has been carried on until final facts or conclusions are distinguished from primal inference, after the monkey and the parrot have both got through, there is brought in a verdict of the whole matter, and this is called judgment. Judgment is that faculty which enables the mind to ascertain truth by comparing facts and ideas. Judgment is the faculty of opinion put by the individual upon facts with which he has become acquainted, and upon ideas which have been generated within his own brain. A judgment having been formed, the will rises and executes the mandates of the judgment. The will is the power of determining upon final action, and upon the will human achievement largely depends.

Now remember that intellectual action of the mind works as follows: First, you have impression through one of the senses; then perception of that impression, that is consciousness; then intuition, then thought, then reasoning, then understanding, then judgment, then will.

Beyond the intellectual workings of the human mind, we have, as a compass to guide the will, what men call conscience. Theodore Parker, when a little boy, was tempted one day to kill a spotted tortoise, but a voice spoke to him and said "It is wrong." He looked around, and seeing no one, fled in great fear to his mother, and told her what he had heard and asked her what it was that spoke to him in that way. The mother took the child in her arms, and said: "Some men call it conscience, but I prefer to call it the voice of God speaking in the soul of man. If you heed that little voice it will always guide you aright."

The will is swayed and impelled, or hindered, by what are called the emotions. The emotions have been subdivided into feelings, and passions. The extremes of feeling are termed pleasure, and pain. These vary through all grades of intensity, from the faintest flush of satisfaction, to the brightness of ecstatic joy; from the slightest cloud of discontent, to the stormiest violence of grief and agony. They intermingle with all the experiences and energies of the mind, intruding upon every affection investigating every movement of the intelligence, and animating or disheartening every activity of the free will. Passions are represented on the one extreme by love, and on the other by hate. When these are but partially developed, we may feel pity, or disgust, or contempt for objects about us.

Emotions are sometimes awakened by the idea that things are true, or beautiful, or good. Such emotions are called the intellectual sense, the æsthetic sense, and the moral sense. Again, the emotions may be excited by the originality or newness of the idea. If new and incongruous, it is known as the emotion of the ludicrous. An emotion when vividly presented in bright language is termed repartee.

Again, the mind is the parent of desires. Some may be normal and healthful, while others are irregular and morbid. Desires belonging to the physical constitution are commonly known as appetites. Healthful appetites, when naturally satisfied, cease their craving, and disappear until the health and well-being of the body reawaken them. Unnatural appetites continue their demands for that which is unhealthy and injurious. The will is not always energetic enough to subdue such appetites. Concerning unnatural appetites, Charles Dickens has declared that "vices are sometimes only virtues carried to excess."

And now, as we rehearse these various and numerous faculties of the mind, we come to the conclusion that the mind is single, yet with a plurality of functions. It is the same mind that feels, that thinks, and that wills; and in putting forth either of these functions it never entirely ceases from the others. Consequently, every mental state has something of feeling, something of intelligence, and something of volition, or endeavour. It is so with the body. The body puts forth simultaneously various functions of animal life. It breathes, it circulates its blood, it digests, it secretes, and it receives, and transmits sensations. Not one of these bodily functions need be suspended while the others are in exercise. The human mind works as a unit. One function may appear temporarily to overshadow by its prominence all others, and yet the other functions are by no means suspended. The various functions of the mind shade into each other with an infinitely varying degree of prominence, and thus give a kaleidoscopic character to the mental states.

It needs but little reflection to conclude that the uses

to which our brains must be subjected are both intricate and multitudinous. They have a priestly charge and oversight over those living temples so "fearfully and wonderfully made" by the hand of Infinite Wisdom; and they are likewise the temporary lodging places of the immortal soul. The brain is the great storehouse of fact and the factory of thought. It takes up by its inherent action the scenes and sounds by which it is surrounded; it gorges itself upon the experiences of the past; it protrudes itself, through hope and imagination, upon the great undiscovered future. Within the serried ranks of cell and fibre, of matter gray and white, there is involved in meshes, too intricate to unravel, a mysterious union of the material and the immaterial. The theories of the wisest are too feeble to express it, the explorations of the ages have failed to discover or explain in full the unfathomable phenomena of mental action. Materialistic theorists find no satisfactory conclusions from their varied and persistent investigations of the human brain and its marvellous workings. From action to inaction, from life to death, the search for the truth has been and is being most carefully made. The brain is the sheltering home of mentality, of immortal being, too, but you might as well count the rafters of a church, and from the enumeration thereof declare the character of the congregation therein assembled, as to attempt to educe from an examination of the brain after death a conclusive theory as to the nature of man. And yet the investigation goes on, and the problem of human life will by-and-by be solved. Gradually the cause and effect of perception, impression, and ratiocination, will be surely evolved.

The practical uses to which our brains are adapted are those of self-preservation and self-improvement. With what critical care, then, should we begin and continue the exercise of that organ upon whose proper development and growth depend the life, the happiness, the prosperity, and progress of the individual possessor of so rare a gift! The young should be taught to regard the brain in their possession as the pearl of great price. Brain culture of the right kind should begin at the earliest possible period in life, and should be continued without undue interruption, until man bends his head low to escape the rafters in the western horizon. This does not mean hard study, but proper training in childhood. Our brains should always be used with moderation and steadiness, but with unswerving persistence. Upon this care and culture depends not only the growth of the individual, but, by such means are fortifications erected to repel the assaults of man's greatest enemy—insanity.

The best uses of the brain are those in which all the forces of that organ are bent to the service of right, and are forever arrayed against the hordes of wrong.

The wost abuse of the brain is a prostitution of its powers before the juggernaut of sin and error. It is a mournful fact that great powers and great abuses are often found in close company. The exercise of these powers, and the exemplification of wrong use are often manifest in the life and career of a single individual, and sometimes they are manifest in the acts of a community, or a nation.

While we recognize the powers and achievements of the human mind, yet we can never see that mind at work. The wisest thought of the philosopher, or the finest conception of the poet, may produce no observable action of the brain. The school boy's determination to run away from school may produce as much effect upon his brain as was produced upon Cæsar's or Napoleon's when one decided to cross the Rubicon, and the other to scale the heights of Saint Bernard. But while we cannot see the actual workings of the human mind, we are yet able to trace in history the effects of those workings. To attempt to measure the work of the brain in civilization would be but an attempt to measure civilization itself. A greater range of mental and moral perceptions, and a superior fineness of mental and moral culture, are really all that have been gained in the centuries of human life. I am speaking, of course, of the permanent possessions of the human mind. What is preserved in the intellectual life of the past in books, pictures, architecture, and sculpture, is an available aid of great value. But apart from this, something has been preserved of the strength and culture which habits of thinking produce, and this is all that man can definitely claim as his own; all else is outside of himself and may be destroyed. But while we all understand, abstractly, that the brain is the seat of intellectual life, and that it impels all human action and shapes all human destiny, yet there are few so well instructed that they would not be filled with surprise and wonder at what one man may do. In mingling with the masses of human beings, the thought impressed most forcibly upon us is the littleness, the insignificance, of an individual life. Count a hundred of those you will first meet on your way tomorrow morning, and the chances are that the world would not feel the slightest loss if they were to be instantly swept out of existence; nor would it lack anything of its intellectual acquisitions if they had never been. What more painful, humiliating illustration of man's littleness! But you *can* count a hundred names whose loss, if they should be taken from civilization, would make immeasurable mutilations. What empty shelves in our libraries; what vacant spaces on the walls of our galleries of art; what grand structures, the inspirations of genius and of faith, would disappear! What rents would be made in laws, in constitutions, in religious creeds! But more impossible to estimate than all else would be the weakening of the intellectual fibre, and the depletion of the intellectual strength, of the living brain. It is by considering these great men whose displacement would wrench the world; it is by studying and trying to measure their work, that we come, in part, to appreciate the capabilities of the human brain. Biography when truthful, and the subject is noble as well as great, is one of the most useful of studies. Nothing else gives us such grand ideas of our nature, such consciousness of strength, such buoyancy of hope, such honorable pride. Nothing else fills us with such longings, or so stirs emulation, and stimulates action; and nothing else imposes upon us more forcibly the importance of correct mental training.

We have pointed out very briefly, some of the normal functions of the brain and mind, in order that we may understand more readily those departures from the normal status which constitute the disease known as insanity. We shall in our next lecture seek to disclose those conditions, and impulses, and forces, which tend to the production of mental disorder; "but that is another story".

Lecture II

THE INSANE DIATHESIS
OR
ABNORMAL TENDENCIES OF THE HUMAN MIND

It has been truly said that "man is the product of his antecedents multiplied by his environments". Our lecture today will concern both of these factors in the sum of human experience.

Dr. Duncan, of Chicago, classifies babies under two heads, —namely, the "acid" and the "alkaline", and from such a physiological standpoint he argues new methods by which our infant population may be best trained in the way it should grow. Dr. Grauvogel, in his metaphysics of medicine, entitled 'The Test Book of Homœopathy", designates the various constitutions of the human body as "hydrogenoid", "oxygenoid", and "carbo-nitrogenoid". As inherent characteristics may be thus classified and designated, why is it not equally legitimate to specify other natural or acquired mental abnormalities by terms of a similar basic import?

Mental abnormality is always due to either imperfect or eccentric physical development, or to effects of inborn or acquired physical disease, or to injurious impressions, either ante-natal or post-natal, upon that delicate and intricate physical structure known as the human brain. Some physical imperfections more than others give rise to mental derangements. Some persons, more than others, when affected by any bodily ailment, tend to aberrated conditions of the mind. Some impressions, more than others, are peculiarly unfortunate by reason of their corroding effects upon the brain tablets of a sensitive mind. To these natural defects and unnatural tendencies, we apply, in a general way, the term "The Insane Diathesis". This is a state or condition in mental pathology corresponding to those diatheses so common in physical pathology, namely, the scrofulous, the cancerous, the scorbutic, the rheumatic, the gouty, and the calculous. The insane diathesis is a general term applying to all those conditions which tend to the inception and growth of mental unsoundness. This diathesis may be either inherited or acquired. In the former case it may be compared to the scrofulous; and in the latter, to the gouty diathesis.

Those who are born to become insane do not necessarily spring from insane parents, or from an ancestory having any apparent taint of lunacy in the blood. But they do receive from their progenitors, oftentimes, certain impressions upon their mental and moral, as well as upon their physical being, which impressions, like iron moulds, fix and shape their subsequent destinies. Hysteria in the mother may develop the insane diathesis in the child. Drunkenness in the father may impel epilepsy, or mania, or dementia, in the son. Ungoverned passions, from love to hate, from hope to fear, when indulged in overmuch by the parents, may unloose the furies of unrestrained madness in the minds of the children. Even untempered religious enthusiasm may beget a fanaticism that cannot be restrained within the limits of reason.

As the development of progress is slow and gradual, so likewise is the development of degeneracy. As men attain high moral and intellectual achievements only through the efforts of succeeding generations, so it seems but natural that the insane should oftentimes trace their sad humiliation and utter unfitness for the duties of life back through a tedious line of passion unrestrained, of prejudice, bigotry, and superstition unbridled, of lust unchecked, and of nerve resource wasted, exhausted, and made bankrupt before its time.

Here are dangers to the human race which potent drugs cannot avert. Here are maladies which medicines cannot cure. But the medical man, the conservator of the public health, realizing the dangers which threaten his community or state, may help, if he will, to parry those pathological blows which the present aims at the future; and, by timely warnings and appeals to his clients of today, may save them for his own treatment, instead of consigning them to an asylum where his own fees cease from doubling, and the crazed ones are at rest.

Causes

Now what are the causes, the outward evidences, of internal degeneracy, and the best means for the prevention of this early beginning, steadily growing, far reaching curse which comes only to torment its victims with purgatorial tortures before the time?

The causes of the insane diathesis are most frequently traceable to the methods of life of those who produce children under such circumstances and conditions that their offspring bear the indelible birthmark of mental weakness. A cause is found in the early dissipations of that father who brings to the work of perpetuating his kind only an exhausted and enfeebled body, and a demoralized and *blasé* mind. A cause is discovered in the mother who contributes her mite to earthly immortality, but who tarnishes that mite with the dross of her own unholy and unhealthy existence. Fast living, such as society in many cases seems to demand, is a fruitful cause of the mental imperfections so common among the rising generation. The sons of royalty, and the sons of the rich, are often weak in cerebral force because of the high living of their ancestry. Many of the high livers of the present day are developing, rapidly and surely, strong tendencies to both mental and physical disorders. Elbert Hubbard says of those who waste their substance upon the Waldorf-Astoria air, that they are apt "to have gout at one end, general paresis at the other, and Bright's disease in the middle".

Causes of the insane diathesis are developed from the parent's unclipped imagination, or sordid desire, or base motive, of succession of mean action, or trial of fear, or passion of remorse, or undue gratification of the appetites, or depletion of the bodily system through over-use, or from any perversion of the physical, mental, or moral powers. The insane diathesis is a product of all those forces which tend to rack and wreck the minds and bodies of those whose lives do not conform to the highest precepts of the laws of nature. It is a "genetic evolution" of the worse from the bad.

"Cursed be the social wants that sin against the strength of youth!"

* * * * * * *

"Cursed be the sickly forms that err from honest nature's rule!!"

Not only is the insane diathesis the fruit of wrong living and wrong thinking in the early lives of the parents, but it is often the result of peculiar states in which the reproducing pair find themselves at the supreme moment of conception; and, likewise, in the unpleasant emotions induced by the surroundings of the mother during pregnancy. Drunkenness, lust, rage, fear, mental anxiety, or even incompatibility, if admitted to participation in the act of impregnation, will, each in turn or in combination, often set the seal of their presence in the shape of idiocy, imbecility, eccentricity, or absolute insanity. The famous Diogenes recognized this fact when he reproached one of those half-witted, crack-brained unfortunates, with the remark: "Surely, young man, thy father begat thee when he was drunk." Burton, in his Anatomy of Melancholy, also states that "If a drunken man gets a child it will never likely have a good brain." And the wise Michelet predicts: "Woe unto the children of darkness, the sons of drunkenness who were, nine months before their birth, an outrage on their mothers." And again: "He who is born of a nocturnal orgy, of the very forgetfulness of love, of a profanation of the beloved one, will drag out a sad and troubled life." The children of drunkards are often sad and hideous burlesques upon normal humanity.

Other unfortunate passions and conditions exert as deleterious effect upon the formative process of new human life as drunkeness. As an example we give the following authentic case: A father had the pleasure of seeing two of his sons grow up strong and vigorous, mentally and physically, while a third was weak, irresolute, fretful, suspicious, and half demented. He confessed to his physicians the cause of this family mishap in these words: "In the summer of 18—I failed, owing to my rogue of a partner running off with all our money. No man perhaps ever felt such a misfortune more keenly than I did, and it seemed to me I should never get over the shock. I was completely unmanned, and feared I should go crazy. Well, during this state of things my wife conceived, and there is the result. Poor S—! He inherits just the state of mind I was then in."

Scores of such cases might be cited. Such warnings are neither single nor singular. Such consequences are the inevitable results of an utter disregard of the simple and plain requirements of nature. A sound body and a cheerful mind can only be produced from healthy stock. Those who multiply, with disease in their bones, care on their minds, and canker in their hearts, simply perpetuate and intensify their own pains and sorrows and cares.

Unpleasant influences brought to bear upon the mother during the period of pregnancy, are marked by a production of a vast variety of mental peculiarities. Historical, scientific, and medical works, are replete with the untimely records. Rizzio was murdered in the presence of his paramour, Mary, Queen of Scots, she being at that time pregnant with James the Sixth. Her son, though a monarch, and born to rule, had a constitutional timidity of temperament, and a great terror of a drawn sword. This was due to the shock of seeing her lover killed while she was pregnant. Ishmael practiced the insanity of hate because his mother lived with that emotion uppermost in her heart while bearing within her body the germ of a nation of haters. The first Napoleon became a great warrior, and cherished the delusion of destiny, because his mother, while carrying him in her womb, "exercised queenly powers over her spirited charger and the subordinates of her huband", and daily associated with the bravest and the best, as well as the most superstitious, of the French army.

Those of you who wish to pursue further the study of the laws of heredity, may do so by consulting the works of Ribot, of Galton, and of Lucas.

Children born under the influence of fear are quite likely to be troubled with apprehensions of impending calamity so intense that they, at last, become insane. Mr. P.—murdered his wife and nine children. Fear pervaded the minds of several pregnant women in the neighbourhood lest they should meet with a similar fate; and the children born soon after grew up to be crazed by the same emotion that had almost paralyzed their feminine progenitors. An insane man always manifested the greatest fear of being killed, and constantly implored those around not to hurt him. His mother had lived with a drunken husband who had often threatened to kill her, once pursuing her with a carving knife. She managed to escape, and shortly afterwards gave birth to this son, who was constantly possessed with the pangs of fear, until he finally took his own life that he might escape apprehended dangers.

Not only individuals, but communities, are sometimes affected by some intense emotion which pervades the minds of all the inhabitants of the country. Esquirol remarks that the children born soon after the horrors of the French Revolution turned out to be weak, irritable, susceptible, and liable to be thrown by the least excitement into insanity. The same may be said of children born during the war in this country, extending from 1861 to 1865.

As we have already stated, the insane diathesis may be acquired as well as inherited, and by the following means:

1. By imperfect nutrition,
2. By slight and almost imperceptible injuries to the brain—blows or falls,
3. By those fears which are sometimes excited in the minds of young children for purpose of government,
4. By overtaxing the undeveloped physical powers,
5. By unwise forcing of the mind in its immature or underdeveloped stage,
6. By premature and unnatural excitement of the sexual organs of the young,
7. By suppression of the ambitions, and powers, and tastes, and desires, of the enthusiastic adolescent.

Insanity is a result of a diseased condition of the brain, either functional or organic, and it manifests itself most frequently by mental disturbance or distress, and by the expression of delusions or hallucinations. It is easy, therefore, to comprehend the fact that whatever tends to the weakening of the cerebrum, or exhaustion of the central forces of life, must necessarily favour the inception and growth of insanity. Lack of proper nutrition for the brain is, then, a prime cause of acquired mental abnormality.

As severe blows upon the head produce immediate and dangerous diseases of the brain which often speedily terminate the lives of those injured, so slight blows, quickly forgotten, perhaps, not infrequently result in stealthily developed, but none the less dangerous, conditions, which eventuate in the derangement of all the mental faculties. There can be no law too severe for the punishment of those who strike children on the head. If you see a parent or teacher boxing the ears of a child, it is your Christian duty to secure his arrest and punishment. He is guilty of slow murder of the innocents. These fiends in human form are the arch-enemies of development and progress.

As fright to the mother, before her child is born, may produce an unfortunate impression upon the offspring, so fright to the young child, occasioned by threats of punishment, by locking up in dark rooms, or by stories of greedy bears or grinning ghosts, produces, oftentimes, a mental shock that makes the child wretched in early life, and drives him into insanity at a later date.

As insanity is most prevalent among the working classes, and as it frequently succeeds utter exhaustion of all physical forces, it follows most conclusively that overwork of the young is a permanent cause of gravitation towards lunacy. Our factories, shops, and stores, not only produce and display artistic and useful wares, but when the young are employed in them, and overtaxed by day and night, they become the feeders of hospitals for the insane, as well as producers of material for premature graves. The regulation by law of the hours during which young operators may work, and the legal limitations which prevent very young persons from working in factories at all, are wise and useful measures for the general welfare of the community. But the effort in this direction should be continued until a proper standard of comfort, and care, and fair treatment, has been established in every working centre.

One of the most common causes of acquired tendency to insanity is the forcing system employed in the education of the young. While we believe that a proper education and training of the human mind is one of the best prophylactics against insanity, we hold also that, like all other agencies which, when misdirected, become the most terrible instruments of evil, the system of popular education, as now practiced in many of our schools and colleges, is fraught with dangers that are likely, unless checked, to destroy the very end it is intended to accomplish.

Instead of seeking, first, to insure a sound physical basis for the mental superstructure, our present methods tend to break down physical health, to dry up the primal sources of existence, and to bring to eventual wreck all the powers of body and of mind. These dangers arise not so much from the amount of work required, as from the amount of anxiety and worry which this work induces in the minds of sensitive children. Many children of the present generation are sensitive, with nervous temperaments, and they are easily affected by the strain of mental toil. Such children should be held in check, or guided by enlightened intelligence, profound wisdom, and ripened judgment, on the part of the teachers. Delicate children should be kept much in the open air, and taught to exercise their muscles until they are fully developed physically. The brain of the child should lie fallow until general physical strength and stamina are insured. Every possible means for developing the physical structure to perfection should be adopted in the training and education of children whose ancestry has been cultivated and refined overmuch from a mental standpoint. Especially should every child be taught to breathe slowly and deeply, and be made to realize the fact that every deep breath of pure air drawn into the lungs adds to the potency of energy, and the prolongation of life.

When our public educators come to appreciate the sublime fact that the human body and the physical brain must be first sufficiently developed and perfected, and that mental growth must be judiciously restrained, and that the minds of the young must be guided in their early achievements with discriminating judgment, then our schools will no longer be hot-beds for the propagation of imbecility, nor gardens for the cultivation of lunatics. Mental culture may accompany physical growth, but always in the order of an army following its leader.

When perfect discipline is attained, and the hour for battling with the world arrives, then the mental forces of those who are physically strong will certainly march to the front, and they will take with them the inspirations of health and good blood. The truant school boy often makes the most successful man because he has insisted upon a proper development of his own physical resources, and in this way he has acted upon his own responsibility.

That grand philosopher, Herbert Spencer, referring to the evils of intellectual cramming, voices a timely warning to both youth and age in these emphatic words: "On old and young the pressure of modern life puts a still increasing strain. Go where you will, and before long there come under your notice cases of children, or youths of either sex, more or less injured by undue study. Here, to recover from a state of debility thus produced, a year's vacation has been found necessary. There you will find a chronic congestion of the brain that has already lasted many months, and threatens to last much longer. Now you hear of a fever that has resulted from the over-excitement in some way brought on at school. And, again, the instance is that of a youth who has already had once to desist from his studies, and who, since he has returned to them, is frequently taken out of his class in a fainting fit."

And again: "How commonly constitutions are thus undermined will be clear to all who, after noting the frequent ailments of hard-worked professional and mercantile men, will reflect on the disastrous effects which undue application must produce upon the undeveloped system of the young. The young are competent to bear neither as much hardship, nor as much physical exertion, nor as much mental exertion as the full-grown. Judge, then, if the full-grown so manifestly suffer from the excessive mental exertion required of them, how great must be the damage which a mental exertion, often equally excessive, inflicts upon the young."

A marked case of imperfect nutrition and mental overwork resulting in insanity came under my notice. The patient, a young ambitious Welshman, was brought up on a farm where he was overworked and indifferently fed. From this hard and monotonous life he passed to the severe study and indoor confinement necessary to preparation for college. Though slight in form and weak in body, he succeeded in his new work remarkably well, and was a leader in intellectual achievements at the academy in his native village. After graduating from the academy he entered college, but only to break down under the unnatural strain;

and in a few weeks he passed from the quiet shades of learning to the shadier refuge of an insane asylum. The diathesis in this case was acquired by the means mentioned, for there is no history of hereditary taint, and no other causes for insanity to be found. Such a case illustrates both the unwisdom of the victim for pursuing such a suicidal course, and the folly of his parents in permitting it to be entered upon by the son. It should also serve as a warning to those who are yet free from the distressing toils of unwise scholarly ambition.

In addition to the dangers of excessive mental strain which beset the young in our present hot-beds of learning, we find a leading and growing tendency to excess in social pleasures. We find that the days are passed in exhausting study, and the nights given over to unrestrained social enjoyments. Business and pleasure should always find a happy and harmonious combination in our daily lives, but the amount of each should be very much reduced in the daily round of the average young American. Excessive athletic sports are likewise dangerous, and produce disastrous consequences upon both the heart and the brain.

Children in schools are not only sometimes overworked, but in some boarding schools they are also very apt to be underfed. Hurried and imperfect feeding on the part of the young should be scrupulously avoided. While you may live happily on very plain and inexpensive food, it should always be carefully and properly cooked. You should secure good, plain, wholesome fare in abundance, if you would succeed as a student. My advice to every young man or woman is to keep his or her stomach full of good nourishing food, and to acquire an education at a slow but systematic pace. Eat apples, oranges, oatmeal porridge, cracked wheat mush, graham bread, fresh eggs, peas and beans, salads and olive oil, and but little meat. The ancients lived to be one hundred and twenty years old with eyes undimmed, and they ate and drank and flourished on "corn, wine, and oil".

Another cause of the insane diathesis lies in premature, improper, and unnatural use of the sexual organs. Many of the hospitals for the insane present histories and marks of this unfortunate habit. Every unnatural use and over-excitement of the sexual organism tends not only to epilepsy, but to imbecility, mania, and dementia. The young should be taught to avoid masturbation because it is a source of much mental weakness and abnormality.

Again, the suppression of ambition, or taste, or desire, leads to disappointment and mental depression in the young. A boy may wish to enter one of the learned professions, or to take up some mercantile pursuit, but through the force of circumstances he may be obliged to engage in some menial toil, and thus a laudable ambition is sacrificed to necessity. A girl may have a taste for music or painting, but the binding and repressing force of poverty may prevent the gratification of such a taste, and this may lead to bitter disappointment and depression of all the mental faculties. The repression of a natural desire may impel its victim to drift into the slough of despond. These subtle causes of mental disorder should be carefully considered, and every commendable impulse of the young should be gratified so far as possible, in order to avoid the pitfall of insanity. There is no country in the world where the possibility of rising to eminence, to fame, and to fortune is so broad, so bright, and so encouraging as in this favored land. And yet there is no country in the world more replete with broken wrecks of disappointed ambition than this. We meet such wrecks in every street and thoroughfare of the great cities, and along the highways and byways of the country. They flock about the tables of the money changers in Wall street; and they hover, like flies, in the neighbourhood of every office or position of honour, political or otherwise, throughout the length and breadth of the several states. When the means used for the gratification of man's ambition fail, when hope deferred has made the heart sick, then there creeps in a mental state and a physical condition which favor most strongly the production and the ripening of insanity. A reasonable ambition is necessary for the accomplishment of every noble task, but that ambition is unwise and unholy, when, under its effects, the young break down and wear out prematurely, and when under its sweeping shock they become disgruntled wrecks which even the gentle ministrations of an insane asylum cannot possibly repair. Moderate ambition will lead to ripe achievement; excessive ambition is worse than the battle path of glory, for it "leads but to the grave" direct, while the former drags its victims through years of weary suffering before the rest of the tomb is vouchsafed to their tired bones.

Now the question arises: What are the outward evidences of the insane diathesis? They are numerous and complicated. They present themselves in every varying shade of imperfect physical development, in endless varieties of cranial contour, and in numerous types of facial expression. To understand them most fully, let us present an historical model of a well-balanced brain; and contrast it with the appearance of one whose tendency is to mental obliquity.

Every one recognizes a healthy constitution and rare mental equipose when the name of the illustrious Washington is mentioned. No one ever suspected the Father of his Country of leanings toward insanity. What regularity invested his every feature! What benevolence and good sense characterized and tempered his expression! He had passions like unto other men; but he likewise possessed wonderful powers of self-control. Undisturbed amid the whirling storms of popular excitement, Washington withstood many shocks before which weaker men would have been swept into the pitfall of insanity. Few men are further removed from inclination to madness than was the immortal Washington.

Contrast the brain symmetry of such a man with the uncanny shapes and illogical action of one whose bent is ever toward that which is incongruous and intellectually dicrotic. Picture the benign features of the first President, and again behold in the description of Dickens the distorted countenance of a Quilp, chattering vengeance against those around him. Contrast the beaming expression of him who was first in his countrymen's hearts with that wretched Barnaby Rudge of whom the master of novelists writes: "He was about three and twenty years old, and though rather spare, of fair height and strongly made. His hair, of which he had a great profusion, hung about his face and shoulders, and gave his restless looks an expression quite unearthly—enhanced by the paleness of his complexion... Startling as his aspect was, there was something plaintive in his wan and haggard looks. *For the absence of the soul is far more terrible in a living man than in a dead one;* and in this unfortunate being its noblest powers were wanting. In his face there was wildness and vacancy."

Had Dickens better understood the mysteries of psychology, he would not have claimed that the soul was absent, but that it found but a faint expression through the unfortunate medium of a soggy and misshapen brain.

In the faces of those whose diathesis is that of a sickly mentality, there are always the marks of disorder and desolation. Their "dome of thought" is but a dilapidated "mansard", and the windows of their souls are darkened from within by an unseemly and non-protective armament against approaching storms.

The heads of those who are born or bred to insanity are almost always misshapen. One side is fuller than the other; one ear is set higher than the other; the eyes peer forth in a restless uncertain way from beneath beetling brows; the nose slants slightly across the fact; the mouth has an uneven cut, and the lips match each other but poorly.

There are also in such persons a great variety of expression—the sinister, the ugly, the mock-sober, the leering, the vacillating, the tricky. There may be developed, unmistakably, in the features of the prospective lunatic the malice of the mule, the cunning of the fox, the grinning fiendishness of the hyena, or the sedate sottishness of swine. All these external marks and appearances are but the mirrored images of distorted minds. Inherent crookedness is thus oftentimes forcibly displayed, and the tendencies of the inner man to wallow in the mire of mental ruin are ever thus revealed.

Are there means for avoiding the development and growth of the insane diathesis? Are there means for the cure or relief of transmitted or acquired mental defects? Here are questions which the generations of the past have left unanswered. Yet the solution of such problems may, I believe, be accomplished.

To avoid the evils liable to arise from the propagation of the insane diathesis, the parties to the crime must pause and study the new philosophy of life—a philosophy which shall guide them to the accomplishment of good and noble results, rather than to those which are ignoble and demoralizing to humanity. The avoidance of debasing passion;

the putting away of that cup whose contents is adder's juice; the shunning of all unnecessary anxiety and cares of life, and in their stead the patient cultivation of all higher virtues and better tempers, will, at last, insure an offspring that will not only bless their ancestry, but will fill the earth with happiness, and health, and contentment of mind and spirit.

"Like begets like" though with increasing or decreasing intensity not only in physical contour, but in mental symmetry or mental idiosyncrasy; and not only are the general thoughts and emotions of the parents impressed upon their children, but even the flitting passion of a moment may cast a cloud of darkness over an entire life, just as the silvered sheet of the photographer receives a fadeless impression from a transient ray of sunlight. The mind of the unborn, like the cylinder that revolves in the phonograph, may receive impressions of happy or unholy thoughts, and reproduce them with faithful accuracy in the years to come; aye! even when the brain of the mother is but dust, and her heart no longer responds to any emotion, and her guiding hand is palsied by the chilling touch of death.

To that "holy of holies" then, the sacred temple of procreation, should be brought only such offerings as are sure to prove acceptable to the Lord of Nature. While the mother bears within her being the helpless new life, there should surround her a magic presence of benign and stimulating influences, from which influences the coming mind may draw inspirations that shall feed and nourish and develop all its forces to a symmetrical perfection.

When once the human being has appeared upon the carpet of life, then the practical work of development and growth should begin. The great end should now be to remedy, as far as possible, all inherent defects, and to promote the growth of all possible virtues and powers. The child should be watched over, and guided, and guarded with the same jealous care that was, or ought to have been, exercised toward the mother during the sacred term of pregnancy. If proper care is taken, the ungainly in body and the weak in mind may develop both symmetry and usefulness. Even in the worse types of mental disease there are some salient and bright spots upon which good influences may act:

> "There is some soul of goodness in things evil.
> Would men observingly distil it out."

Bright surroundings, pleasant associations, stimulating encouragements, abundant food of the best and plainest quality, fresh air, active exercise, in the clear sunlight, together with simple direction not forcing of the mental faculties, will, in the course of patient time, produce from ever poor stock such a robust and cultured race as to be the astonishment of those who furnish and mold the material.

In making these marches to higher and better things, we may, I think, be permitted to state that homœopathy has already done much, and will do more, with the medicines at her command. Medicine may not only cure active disease, but, if properly applied, it may act as a stimulus in the growth and development of the human body. Such remedies as Calcarea Carbonica, and Hepar Sulphur, and Graphites, and Phosphorus, and Sepia, and Silicea, and Sulphur, have here a field of action surpassing any in which they have heretofore wrought. The "tissue remedies", so-called, are, we believe, destined to win triumphs in this new arena, which shall transcend all the glories of medical achievement in the past. God hasten the day when we may learn how to wield aright these mighty weapons against fateful heredity and acquired degeneracy!

In conclusion, we offer another warning and another injunction to the young, to the effect that not only must the mental powers be protected from premature exhaustion by overwork, but they must also be fortified against the too common dissipations of youth, and sustained by the recuperative influences of timely and abundant sleep. It is natural to be spendthrift of those gifts which have been lavishly bestowed upon us, and of which we seem to have an exhaustless supply. Hence we waste our youthful vigor, amid scenes of exciting folly, not only by day, but through the long-drawn and precious hours of the night—hours that are precious because of their designed purpose to replenish and restore the inevitable wastes of life. Through moderation alone are happiness and health long-conserved. The midnight lamp of the worker, and the midnight lamp of the pleasure seeker, alike consume with undue avidity the cruse of oil alloted to each one's life. Therefore the lamp must be put out early if the owner would live long and well in the land.

Not only must excessive waste be shunned, but restoration and repair must be steadily and perseveringly attained. The sin of omission is quite as heinous as the sin of commission. To neglect the maintenance of one's powers, in their fullest possible measure, is as deplorable and wrong as the throwing away of strength already acquired.

The precepts embodied in such experiences and such teachings as we have endeavored to trace in this lecture are, we believe, sound and practical. If the medical profession would rise to the duty of properly warning both the young and their natural guardians, and if these would give heed to such warnings, then the incomputable evils of premature forcing of the brain would be averted; the folly of dissipation would be shunned, the necessity for ceaseless repair would be recognized, and the sources of mental unsoundness, now burdened with a tropical luxuriousness, would become barren and unproductive as the sullen shores of the dark Dead Sea.

Lecture III

SLEEP, SLEEPLESSNESS, AND THE CURE OF INSOMNIA

Today we shall seek to discuss the nature and quality of sleep—Sleep, "the twin sister of Death". We shall also portray the necessity for sleep, and nature's method for securing it. Again, we shall consider the causes of sleeplessness; and finally, we shall endeavor to point out the safest and surest dietetic, medical, and other means for the cure or relief of insomnia.

Some of you have already learned that sleeplessness is one of the prime and leading indications of approaching insanity. Still, there are many exceptional cases of insomnia which do not terminate in mental unsoundness. But insomnia is so often the forerunner of mental disorder, that it seems proper to devote one lecture of the course on mental disorders to a consideration of sleep and sleeplessness.

Probably no writer in ancient or modern times has so fully discussed the subjects of somnia and insomnia as the immortal Shakespeare. Hence, when we would know of sleep and sleeplessness—of the beneficial effects of the one, and the distressing qualities of the other, we naturally turn for information to the luminous pages of the most wonderful polychrest thinker that the world has ever produced. When we go back to the days of the Bard of Avon, we find from him who "held the mirror up to nature" that many a time and oft the "fring'd curtains of his eyes were all the night undrawn". Shakespeare recorded his own experience as well as that of the men and women who lived in his time.

The sleep of age and of youth is described when Friar Laurence says:

> "Care keeps his watch in every old man's eye,
> And where care lodges, sleep can never lie;
> But where unbruised youth with unstuff'd brain
> Doth couch his limbs, there golden sleep doth reign."

The tranquillity of sleep is outlined here:

> "And to conclude, the shepherd's homely curds,
> His cold thin drink out of his leather bottle,
> His wonted sleep under a fresh tree's shade,
> All which secure and sweetly he enjoys,
> Are far beyond a prince's delicates."

Worry is one of the great causes of sleeplessness:

> "O polish'd perturbation! Golden care!
> That keep'st the ports of slumber open wide
> To many a watchful night! Sleep with it now!
> Yet not so sound, and half so deeply sweet,
> As he, whose brow with homely biggin bound,
> Snores out the watch of night."

The best cause of sleep is honestly acquired fatigue from active exercise:

> "Weariness
> Can snore upon the flint; when restive sloth
> Finds the down pillow hard."

The tired boy sleeps better than the monarch:

> "Canst thou, O partial Sleep, give thy repose
> To the wet sea boy in an hour so rude,
> And in the calmest and most stillest night,
> With all appliances and means to boot,
> Deny it to a King? Then, happy low, lie down!
> Uneasy lies the head that wears a crown."

SLEEP, SLEEPLESSNESS AND THE CURE OF INSOMNIA 43

The golden qualities of sleep are such as to become blessings and benisons from friends to friends:

> "Sleep, Richmond, sleep in peace and wake in joy.
> Thou quiet soul, sleep thou a quiet sleep."

This was Romeo's invocation to Juliet:

> "Sleep dwell upon thine eyes; peace in thy breast."

The goodness of Lady Mortimer is set forth when the poet declares:

> "She will sing the song that pleaseth thee,
> And on thy eyelids crown the god of sleep."

Titania to her lover says:

> "I'll give thee fairies to attend on thee,
> And they shall fetch thee jewels from the deep,
> And sing, while thou on pressed flowers dost sleep."

In behalf of fallen heroes, Titus said:

> "There greet in silence, as the dead are wont,
> And sleep in peace, slain in your country's wars."

Also the poet declares that in that land of the blest there

> "Are no storms,
> No noise, but silence and eternal sleep."

A lack of sleep is the most horrible of earthly terrors:

> "No sleep close up that deadly eye of thine,
> Unless it be while some tormenting dream
> Affrights thee with a hell of ugly devils."

> "Sleep shall neither night nor day
> Hang upon his pent-house lid;
> He shall live a man forbid."

> "Not poppy nor mandragora.

> Nor all the drowsy syrups of the world,
> Shall ever medicine thee to that sweet sleep
> Which thou own'dst yesterday."

The blessings of sleep, on the other hand, are further outlined as follows:

> "With him above
> To ratify our work, we may again
> Give to our tables meat, sleep to our nights."

> "How sweet the moonlight sleeps upon that bank."

> "The best of rest is sleep."

> "Our little lives are rounded with a sleep."

These quotations from the dramas and tragedies of Shakespeare, illustrate the fact that history repeats itself, and that the experiences of humanity are much the same through all the centuries.

Sleep is a prime and urgent necessity of our natures. To secure it in abundance, with system and regularity, is the aim of the philosopher, the dream of the poet, and the easy accomplishment of the workingman. The natural conclusion is that we should all utilize a portion of our time by building railroads, or by digging canals, or, like Gladstone, by chopping down trees.

What is sleep? We are told that "it consists of a temporary suspension of the functions of the cerebral portions of the nervous system." Sleep is the act of closing the doors of the brain against external intrusion while the process of rest and repair is going on within.

The process by which sleep is induced is that of a moderate anemia, or lessened blood supply to the brain. This anemia, while sufficient to quiet the ordinary operations of the mind, is not far enough advanced to restrict the processes of repair in the brain. The theory of cerebral anemia during sleep is supported by the experiments of Alexander Fleming, the investigations of Durham, and the observations of the state of the retina during sleep with the ophthalmoscope by Hughlings-Jackson. Fleming tried compression of the carotid arteries, and succeeded in causing sleep. Durham removed the skull-cap from dogs, and noted that in these animals, when asleep, the brain was always anemic. Hughlings-Jackson found that the expansions of the optic nerve are paler and less congested during sleep than at other times.

Not only is the brain less fully supplied with blood during sleep, that is, not only is the volume decreased, but the velocity with which it flows is likewise diminished. The heart's action is slower and less active during sleep than during wakefulness.

A hyperemic condition of the brain stimulates the greatest mental activity, unless the hyperemia passes to a state of over-powering congestion, while the anemic state promotes rest and repair. The condition for sleep is that of cerebral anemia.

Now what are some of the natural causes of sleep? What are the causes which prevent sleep, and by what means shall the latter be removed? The favoring causes of sleep are the darkness of night, the removal of all disturbing agencies, the horizontal position of the body, an easy and comfortable bed, cessation from toil and thought, a sufficient nourishment to satisfy the demands of the entire system, and a release of the brain from sensorial impressions.

Under these favouring causes the approach of sleep is usually swift and easy. It is said that the mind is "pervaded by a strange confusion which amounts almost to a mild delirium; the ideas dissolve their connection with the mind one by one, and its own essence becomes so vague and diluted that it melts away in the nothingness of slumber".

Health of body and peace of mind are the normal conducements to sleep. Hence we find that the young, the innocent, the healthy, and the happy are the best and most natural sleepers.

Among the assisting causes of sleep, we may name monotonous sounds, such as slow music, the humming of bees, the falling of rain, the rattle of wagons, the roll of street cars, the roar of water-falls, the splash of the ocean surf, and, most of all, the voice of a dull preacher who, armed with a soporific sermon, seems to have no other aim except to put to sleep both the pillars and the gods! Monotonous sounds attract the attention of the mind from inward cares or outward irritation, and lull the senses to narcotic forgetfulness, like the crooning voice of a motherly old nurse.

We may also note, as a sleep producer, the effect of cold upon the system, which promotes, at first, drowsiness, and sometimes an irresistible tendency to sleep. And again, excessive heat tends to indolent inactivity of the body, drowsiness of the mind, and an inclination to doze and slumber. Alcohol, opium, and other drugs are often sleep-compelling when given in overmastering doses. A lymphatic temperament favors likewise the induction of sleep.

Now in considering the causes which prevent sleep, we name:

1. Those pathological conditions of the brain which derange the normal action of the mind. Chief among these are hyperemia, or excessive blood supply, on the one hand, and excessive anemia, or lack of supply, on the other.

2. Protracted overuse of the brain—that is, overwork

until the strain produces, or tends to produce, vasomotor paralysis.

3. Worry. Worry is an undue anxiety over the common or little every-day affairs of life. It is this everlasting worry that produces more than three-fourths of all the mental disasters which befall the children of men. My advice to you is to clean out the sand of worry from the bearings of your existence, and pour in the oil of peaceful contentment with your lot. Then you will run the race of life easily, without danger of friction, or overwear, or hindering hot-boxes on the baggage car of your brain. You may work and study with great vigor during the day, and no harm may result; but when worry finds its way into every recess of reason, when it breaks the back of our better judgment, and stuns our wills, then our brains lose their best powers, and our trains of thought fall into abject and hopeless ruin.

4. The natural temperament of some people is a formidable obstacle to the acquirement of sleep. Bilious people are apt to be melancholy. The nervous temperament impels its owner to rapid action, until exhaustion, irritability, and sleeplessness follow. Victims of an unfortunate temperament seek matrimonial alliances with those who are directly their opposites. The despairing and the despondent should consort with the sunny and the sanguine, while the irritable and excitable should secure, if possible, mates who are lymphatic and placid.

5. Localized disease in some portion of the body, other than the brain, may, by reflex action, produce sleeplessness. Thus we may have disease of the heart, which induces wakefulness. The lungs, the stomach, the liver, the bowels, or the genital organs may all become, through disease and by reflex action, centers of sleep disturbing tendencies. To

cure sleeplessness under such circumstances requires a cure of the organs involved.

We now offer a few practical suggestions for the induction of satisfactory sleep:

1. We should cherish, so far as possible, a philosophical frame of mind. That is, we should "take no thought for the morrow". You should impress this philosophy upon your sleepless patients.

2. To secure sleep we must put the body in proper condition, and this end is attained by proper toil or exercise, by suitable diet, by careful attention to all the excretory organs, and by polishing up the human temple along the line suggested by the old adage: "Cleanliness is next to godliness." He who works and washes wisely and well rarely fails to attain good sleep at night. Before retiring to sleep the bladder and the bowels should be relieved of their contents, if necessary, otherwise they act as localized irritants which, by reflex influence, disturb sleep.

3. Proper nourishment of the body is essential to the acquirement of sleep. If the brain is weak and anemic—that is, below the health level—it must be strengthened and nourished by appropriate nutriment before good sleep can be attained. Thus it happens that a weakly person is often made to sleep well by drinking considerable quantities of hot milk, or beef tea, or some mildly stimulating broth, or soothing gruel, a short time before the hour for sleep arrives. The hungry nerves having been satisfied, sleep comes easily. On the other hand, if there is a tendency to hyperemia of the brain, and an over-active state of the mind, benefit is often derived from partaking of a little plain solid food just before retiring. While the stomach is busy digesting this solid food, the brain may be relieved of engorgement to such an extent as to admit the inception of sleep.

As a rule, in this climate, it is neither safe nor healthful to go to bed on an empty stomach. Of course if a person is a dyspeptic, and subject to much pain during the process of digestion, care should be exercised as to the variety and quality of the food consumed. Individual idiosyncrasies should be considered, and that food should be selected which experience has shown to be the most agreeable and satisfying. Try to find for each individual case the food which most surely agrees, and try to keep your patients away from that food which disagrees. Sometimes if the stomach is very weak, and the mind also, a little good old wine may be taken with the food the last thing at night. Sometimes brandy has a marked influence in the relief of insomnia. Some years ago we had a woman patient who had suffered with intense insomnia for years. We tried various remedies without success. At length we gave her from two to four ounces of brandy each night on going to bed. The patient began to sleep regularly and sufficiently, and in three months the insomnia of years had entirely passed away. The patient slept well, ate well, and became strong and cheerful. As soon as the natural tendency to sleep was restored, the brandy was stopped, but good health and abundant sleep continued.

4. A warm bath, followed by a cold douche and brisk rubbing, will oftentimes produce drowsiness and ability to sleep by those who have been pressed with cares, and who have been irritated or disturbed during the day in body and mind. Business men who are shut up in close offices all day, and who work very hard with their brains, may be greatly relieved by a quick hot and cold bath, followed by a brisk rubbing, just before going to bed. The rubbing should be performed by an attendant, in order to avoid causing extra fatigue to the patient.

5. Fresh air should be supplied freely in every sleeping-room, yet the sleeper should be protected from even moderate draughts; for these, if long-continued, will produce chilliness of one portion of the body, while another portion may be over-heated, and thus a disturbing inequality of circulation ensues.

6. Beds should be firm in texture, level, and well-elevated from the floor; for thus the sleeper is above dangerous, heavy gases. Some think it is wise to have the head toward the north and the feet toward the south, in order that the magnetic currents may affect the system favorably. Bed clothing should be light and porous as practicable. Soft woollen blankets are best. Stiffly starched counterpanes are objectionable, and should be removed at night, because they do not favor good ventilation.

7. The position of the head is of importance during sleep. In cases of hyperemia the head and shoulders should be well elevated by means of large pillows. In cases of anemia, where the heart's action is weak, and the blood supply is imperfect, a very slight elevation should be granted. One small pillow is generally enough for anemic patients.

8. Another means for inducing sleep is massage, or muscular manipulation. This should be applied by a trained nurse, and according to systematic rules, as laid down by the attending physician. If you want to learn more about massage, read Dr. S. Wier Mitchell's interesting work, entitled "Fat and Blood".

We come now to the use of remedies for sleeplessness, and by way of episode we will give you a few ancient prescriptions for the production of sleep. Lemnius advises that you anoint your temples with virgin wax at the hour of sleep. Mizaldus tells us to rub our weary and sleepless brows with rose water and vinegar, together with an ointment made of nutmegs grated upon rose cake, and this to be wet with a little woman's milk. Cardan suggests that we smear our teeth at bed-time with ear wax from a dog. To these may be added oil of nenuphar, wormwood, mandrake, pillows of roses, fat of a dormouse, swine's gall, hare's ears, violet leaves, lovage waters, and *lac virginale*. It seems to me that the application of these remedies should be left to the tastes of the patient!

An ancient and likewise a modern and very valuable remedy for sleeplessness is the common lettuce which grows in every garden. You remember that Venus, after the death of Adonis, her lover, threw herself upon a bed of lettuce in the back yard, and thus gained sleep and forgetfulness of her sorrow. Galen, one of the fathers of medicine, relates that his own sleeplessness was relieved by eating lettuce salad at night.

Upon the principle that a physician, especially a homœopathic physician (who is a physician plus a homœopath), cannot know too much, we present a brief list of old school hypnotics, with the doses, and the authority for their use:

Drug	*Dose*	*Authority*
Bromide of Potash,	5 grs. to 1 dr.,	S. O. L. Potter
Bromide of Soda,	5 grs. to 1 dr.,	,,
Bromide of Calcium,	5 grs. to 1 dr.,	,,
Bromidia,	1 fl. dr. in water,	Battle & Co., St. Louis
Chloral,	2 to 30 or more grs.	Potter
Codeine,	$1/_6$ to 1 gr.,	S. O. L. Potter, Brannan
Bromal Hydrate,	1 to 3 grs., at bed-time,	Dr. Steinauer
Hyoscinæ Hydrobromas,	$1/_{100}$th to $1/_{60}$th gr.,	Potter & Dr. Lyon
Monobromide of Camphor,	1 to 10 grs. in emulsion,	Potter
Morphine,	$1/_{20}$th to ½ gr.,	,,
Opium, powder,	¼th to 2 grs.	,,
Opium, Tincture,	2 minims to 22 drops—1 gr. opium,	

Drug	Dose	Authority
Paraldehyde,	30 minims to 1 dr.	Potter & Granger
Sulfonal, 15 grs. repeated	2 to 5 hours,	Granger, Seguin & Brannan
Trional,	15 to 30 grs.	Henry Morris, M.D.

Probably Sulfonal is one of the most commonly used, and perhaps one of the least harmful hypnotics in general use among our old school brethren of today. It is well to know something of these hypnotics, because you may be called upon to treat patients who have been heavily dosed with them, and you should know what to expect, and how to antidote the effects of such drugs. In our treatment of more than five thousand insane persons, many of whom have suffered with insomnia, we have never felt obliged to use old school remedies in old school doses.

We now give a list of homœopathic remedies, together with the official doses, as prescribed for their physiological effects:

Drug	Dose		Authority
Avena Sativa,	5 to 30 drops,	θ	Dr. Trowbridge
Belladonna,	1 to 30 drops,	θ	Dr. Potter
Cannabis Indica,	5 minims to 1 dr.,	θ	,,
Cimicifuga,	15 minims to 1 dr.,	θ	,,
Coca,	½ to 50 dr., fluid extract,		,,
Coffea,	10 to 50 drops,	θ	Dr. Potter
Gelsemium,	10 drops to 1 dr.	θ	,,
Hyoscyamus,	2 dr. to 1 oz.,	θ	,,
Kali Bromide,	5 grs. to 1 dr.		,,
Moschus,	10 grs. med. dose,		U. S. Dispensatory
Nux Vomica,	1 to 5 or 10 minims,		Dr. Potter
Passiflora,	30 to 40 drops,	θ	Boericke & Tafel
Stramonium,	5 minims to ½ dr.,	θ	Dr. Potter
Valerian,	½ to 2 dr.,		,,
Zincum Met.	1x to 3x,		Dr. Hughes

SLEEP, SLEEPLESSNESS, AND THE CURE OF INSOMNIA 53

We come now to present, as a climax, the characteristic indications for a few of the most prominent homœopathic remedies for sleeplessness. These remedies have been proved, and their symptoms have been duly recorded. We prescribe them in accordance with the "totality of symptoms", and according to the methods laid down by Samuel Hahnemann. The application of these homœopathic remedies affords, we believe, the best results in the long run, and they leave the patient at the end of a course of treatment without injury or damage. We give drop doses once in from one to four hours, according to the severity of the symptoms; and we use the third, sixth, twelfth, and higher potencies. Sometimes we begin with the third decimal, and sometimes with the third centesimal, and go up accordingly.

Aconite.—Sleeplessness after exposure to cold winds, and where there is a full, strong, quick pulse, with great restlessness, anxiety, and fear of death. It may be used in mental anxiety caused by the shock of bad news. (Also Gelsemium, Ignatia, and Opium). Cases of acute melancholia with agitation, or acute mania with great excitability, are often relieved at the outset by the use of Aconite.

Belladonna.—Sleeplessness, with flushed face, dilated pupils, and throbbing in the head. The patient has horrible dreams, from which he awakens in a fright, but he soon overcomes this fright, and becomes hot and pugilistic.

Chamomilla.—Sleeplessness on account of severe pain, such as toothache. The patient is cross and irritable, and inclined to growl and move about. Chamomilla is both ugly and contemptible.

Cimicifuga (Actea Racemosa).—Sleeplessness after drinking, opium eating, and great muscular exertion; after protracted watching, where there is restlessness, and great tremulousness of the muscles throughout the entire system.

Pain in the base of the brain, extending to neck and shoulders. The mind is wrapped in the blackness of eternal darkness. (Some prefer the alkaloid, Macrotin for drunkards and opium eaters. As an antidote to the opium habit, give Macrotin in the third decimal trituration, a two-grain powder every three hours.)

Coffea.—Sleeplessness from excessive mental activity. Excessive sensitiveness to all impressions; fidgety, and cannot compose the mind to sleep. It is best to give Coffea in the sixth or the thirtieth potency.

Gelsemium.—Sleeplessness from nervous irritation, or acute disorders of the nervous system. The patient is dull and stupid, but unable to sleep. Gelsemium is often useful in the sleeplessness of acute alcoholics. Drop doses of the second or third decimal is frequently effective, although sometimes the tincture is administered in two or three drop doses. You may give Gelsemium for acute drunks, for long drunks Nux Vomica and Cimicifuga, and for very long drunks Opium; and when the drunk has continued until great exhaustion, emaciation, and restlessness follows, then give Arsenicum.

Hyoscyamus.—Sleeplessness without apparent cause. The patient is very nervous; jumps in his sleep, and thus awakens himself. While the Hyoscyamus patient cannot sleep, he is nevertheless good-natured and jolly, although inclined to talk upon salacious subjects, and to uncover the body. Women especially when needing Hyoscyamus take off their clothes because they are erotic. The difference between erotomania and nymphomania is this: Erotomania has great mental excitement upon sexual subjects; nymphomania has intense physical desire for sexual intercouse. Both are affected in body and mind, but in the Hyoscyamus case the mental symptoms predominate, while in the physical case Cantharis is called for. Where the patient awakens many times during the night, but falls asleep easily, give Phosphorus. Hyoscyamus has a jolly delirium, Nux Vomica has an intense crossness and irritability, while Phosphorus is sad and solemn.

Kali Bromidum.—This is a valuable remedy for insomnia where it is induced by the exhaustions and irritations of long-continued disease. Large doses of this drug are unnecessary. We use the first decimal trituration, giving a one or two-grain dose every hour during the evening, say from six to eleven o'clock. It is very effective in the sleeplessness of sick and wasted women.

Nux Vomica.—This is suitable for those who sleep during the middle of the night, but awaken about three in the morning. Such cases are usually hard workers, and perhaps hard drinkers. Sometimes they are studious and sad, and sometimes they are lazy, as well as irritable. The Nux Vomica patient rarely comes out of his sullen mood, except to make trouble for others.

Stramonium.—The Stramonium patient is sleepless because he has horrible hallucinations of sight. He sees all kinds of strange animals coming toward him from every direction, and these apparitions produce in his mind a horrible, abject, and cowardly fear which prevents sleep. Stramonium is often called for in the sleeplessness of acute mania and acute alcoholism.

Veratrum Album.—This is a remedy which assists in the induction of sleep where the patient is suffering with acute mania, or puerperal mania, or religious excitement. There is great restlessness of the mind, with pallor of the countenance, coldness of the body, and tendency to collapse of all the vital forces. The patient may be full of religious supplication, or may dream of robbers, or of being bitten by a dog, or of being drowned.

There are a few new remedies for sleeplessness which are sometimes valuable, and generally harmless. Avena Sativa (the common oat) is useful for the sleeplessness of those who are over-worn by hard work until they cannot sleep. The usual dose is fifteen or twenty drops of Avena tincture taken at bed-time. Coca Erythroxylon is sometimes used in neurasthenic, neuralgic, and hysterical cases. Pisidia (the Jamaica dogwood) is another remedy which may be used in behalf of weak, exhausted and sleepless patients. It is sometimes useful in the early stage of acute mania. Passiflora Incarnata is a remedy which has been used with success in the sleeplessness of women who are suffering with great stress of excitement, and who are inclined to break away from their guardians, and to commit suicide.

The subject of sleep is one of vast importance. The condition of sleeplessness is so deplorable as to stimulate not only our sympathy, but our best efforts for its relief. We can do this if we secure the confidence of our clients, and then patiently and perseveringly toil in their behalf. We should give up over-mastering hypnotics, and use homœopathic remedies instead. We should banish morphine from the bedroom of the sleepless, and introduce hot milk instead. We should remember that beyond the temporary relief afforded by large doses of hypnotics, we may find safety and efficacy in

> "Many simples operative
> Whose power will close the eye of anguish."

That was a wise injunction of Meander when he declared that "sleep is the natural cure of all diseases". To be so, however, it must be induced by mind, and not by savage measures. "Let us, then, cultivate sleep—not the sleep of sloth and inertia, not the listless reverie of ennui, not the keff of the Arab or the noonday siesta of the tropics, but that other and nobler Somnus, whose temple, opening only at nightfall, invites the weary, day-worn traveller to rest. Here, with the silent stars for his everlasting ministers, he sits enthroned in halls of sweet obliviousness, waiting with the lavish and impartial affection of a parent, to crown us all with the poppy wreaths of sleep."

Lecture IV

HISTORY AND CLASSIFICATION OF INSANITY

Theories, Definitions, and Forms of Commitment

We shall speak today, very briefly, of the history of insanity, and also give some classifications of this disease, together with theories and definitions. Again, we shall speak of the legal forms of commitment to hospitals for the care of the insane, and advise you when to commit and when to refrain from so doing.

The earliest reference to insanity is found in the book of Deuteronomy. There the Lord, through Moses, makes promises to those who are good, and threats against those who are bad; and among other visitations we note: "So thou shalt be mad for the sight of thine eyes which thou shalt see." Again, we find in Samuel, concerning David: "And he changed his behaviour before them and feigned himself mad in their hands, and scrabbled on the doorposts of the gate, and let his spittle fall down upon his beard." That was a cunning and successful feigning of insanity. Feigning insanity, under distressing circumstances, has been one of the achievements of mankind throughout the centuries. Again, in Ecclesiastes: "I said of laughter, it is mad; and of mirth, what doeth it?" This is a fair description of the condition known as dementia. The preacher also says: "Surely oppression maketh a wise man mad." Here is another ancient but eternal truth, for oppression, if long-continued, is a well-known cause of insanity. Jeremiah declares, concerning the wine cup: "And they shall drink and be moved and be mad." And concerning religious matters, he says: "For every man that is mad and maketh himself a prophet, that thou shouldst put him in prison, and in the stocks." And once more: "They are mad upon their idols." In these statements of priest, prophet, and psalmist, we learn something of the causes and conditions of insanity.

Not only individuals but nations were poisoned by the wine cup in ancient times, for Jeremiah also says: "Babylon has been a golden cup in the Lord's hands, that made all the earth drunken. The nations have drunken of her wine, therefore the nations are mad." It is a universal fact that unwise and intemperate use of any of the blessings of life brings inevitable retribution. On the other hand, the temperate enjoyment of those things which the Creator has made possible is the best way to live.

Greek writers speak of cases of mental aberration as occurring with some frequency in Greece. The inhabitants of the Roman Empire, from the crazy king Nero to the humblest citizen, were afflicted with mental unsoundness; and in ancient Egypt we find that the Egyptians had temples and priests for the care of the insane.

Hippocrates, who flourished about four hundred years before Christ, was the first physician who seemed to have any true conception of the real nature of insanity. He believed that to a certain extent insanity was due to physical disturbances, and yet for many centuries later the masses believed that madness was simply a visitation of the devil.

In the time of Christ the insane were permitted to wander at large among the woods and in the caves of Palestine. Six centuries after Christ, the monks of Jerusalem built the first hospital or asylum for the care of the insane. A century later the fame of St. Dymphna had extended over Europe, from the little village of Gheel, in Belgium, and those afflicted with mental diseases were taken to her shrine for the purpose of being cured.

You will remember that St. Dymphna was an Irish princess who resisted the assaults of an unnatural father, and fled to Belgium, where she engaged herself in the care of the sick. Her father pursued her, and found her, and cut off her head in one of the streets of Gheel. Two insane persons saw the blood gush from her neck, and the shock immediately cured them of their insanity. From that time on St. Dymphna became the patron saint of mental invalids, and the example of her purity of life has been an invisible but potent power for the restoration of the insane from that day to this.

In the year 1409 a hospital for the insane was established at Valencia, in Spain. In the year 1547, the hospital of Saint Mary of Bethlehem was established near London. This institution was known as "Bedlam" for a long time, a name notorious in the history of London.

The first asylum established upon reform principles was St. Luke's in London. This was founded in 1751. About the year 1791, Samuel Hahnemann, the expounder of homœopathy, established an asylum for the insane at Georgenthal, near Gotha, and in this institution the law of kindness was the unvarying rule. Hahnemann, in his "Lesser Writings," says: "I never allow any insane persons to be punished by blows or other corporeal infliction." About 1792 or '93, Pinel struck the chains from the incarcerated insane at the Bicêtre, near Paris.

During the past century there has been a gradual tendency toward better things in behalf of those afflicted with mental disease. A hundred years ago they were treated with prison surroundings and prison fare. Then asylum treatment began to prevail. This is a higher grade of treatment than that bestowed by the prison. Asylum care means close confinement, good food, sufficient clothing, and comfortable beds. Asylum care means the humane custody of dangerous prisoners. From the asylum we move on to the hospital system of caring for the insane. The hospital system recognizes the fact that the lunatic is a sick man, and needs nursing and medical treatment in order to effect a cure. Hospital treatment has been gradually introduced during the past twenty years or more, and in time it will eventually supersede asylum treatment, and prison or workhouse methods in the management of the insane everywhere.

Classification of Insanity

We come now to a classification of insanity. Many classifications have been made. We wish to present to you that which is as brief and simple as possible, hence we make the list as follows:

1. Melancholia, which includes all forms of mental depression,
2. Mania, which includes all forms of mental excitement,
3. Dementia, which includes all forms of mental weakness or failure, except idiocy and imbecility,
4. General paresis, which is a distinct form of mental disease possessing certain characteristics which demand that it shall be classified separately. In general paresis you will find conditions of mental depression, mental excitement, and mental weakness; and in the course of this fatal disease you will find that it embodies and embraces some elements of all other forms of insanity.

We present herewith two classifications. One is known as the British classification, and the other as the American classification.

BRITISH CLASSIFICATION

I. Congenital, or infantile mental deficiency. Idiocy; Imbecility; Cretinism: (*a*) With epilepsy; (*b*) Without epilepsy.

II. Epilepsy acquired.

III. General Paralysis of the Insane

IV. Mania
- Acute
- Chronic
- Recurrent
- A potu, or mania of drunkenness
- Puerperal
- Senile

V. Melancholia
- Acute
- Chronic
- Recurrent
- Puerperal
- Senile

VI. Dementia
- Primary
- Secondary
- Senile
- Organic, i.e., from tumors, hemorrhages, etc.

VII. Delusional Insanity (Monomania)
VIII. Moral Insanity

AMERICAN CLASSIFICATION

I. Mania
- Acute
- Chronic
- Recurrent
- Puerperal

II. Melancholia
- Acute
- Chronic
- Recurrent
- Puerperal

III. Primary Delusional Insanity, Monomania, Subacute Mania (Paranoia?)

IV. Dementia
- Primary
- Secondary
- Organic (tumors, hemorrhages, etc.)

V. General Paralysis of the Insane (General Paresis).

VI. Epilepsy (with Mania or Dementia)

VII. Toxic Insanity (Alcoholism, Morphinism, etc.)

VIII. Congenital or subsequent mental deficiency
- Idiocy
- Imbecility
- Cretinism

These classifications are somewhat more elaborate than the one which I have presented to you, and perhaps this elaboration is necessary in making up an extensive work upon the subject. They are probably serviceable to alienists, but for the general practitioner it may be well to get firmly fixed in mind the four general divisions of insanity—namely, melancholia, mania, dementia, and general paresis,—and hold to them as starting points for wider study and further investigation.

THEORIES

There are three theories concerning the nature of insanity:

1. The ancients believed that insanity was a possession of the devil,—a perversion of the psychical forces through the effects of sin or crime.

2. It is believed by some that insanity is a disease of both body and mind, or that the physical and spiritual forces are both degenerated when under the influence of insanity. If the spiritual forces are immortal, they can never become diseased.

3. The last and most modern theory is, that insanity is a departure from the normal mental status, as a result of diseased conditions of the brain. In other words, insanity is a physical disease, or, at least, all mental aberrations are dependent upon either functional or organic diseases of the brain and nervous system. These conditions of the brain are due, we believe, to disordered blood. The blood is always perverted in insanity. It is either too thin or too thick, and its quality and distribution have been impaired before diseased conditions of the brain are likely to occur.

For general purposes, it is well to remember that the ancients thought insanity to be a diseased condition of the soul, while modern alienists believe that insanity is due to a physical disorder. Between these two extremes there may be many shades of belief, but it is unnecessary to touch upon them at this time. It is essential for the cure of insanity that its physical nature should be recognized, in order that we may deal with it just as we do with any oher physical disease. If you can convert a diseased brain and a diseased body into a sound and healthy brain and body, then you will be likely to have a sound mind as the occupant of the healthy human temple.

Definitions

Dr. Andrew Combe declares insanity to be a "prolonged departure, without an adequate external cause, from the states of feeling and modes of thinking usual to the individual when in health. This is the true feature of disorder

HISTORY AND CLASSIFICATION OF INSANITY

in mind." A general definition of mental disorder is this: Insanity is a departure from the normal mental status of the individual, and this departure is due to some diseased condition of the brain or nervous system. Of course there may be temporary departures from the normal mental status, as when an individual gets drunk, and becomes hilarious, or delirious, or besotted, or stupid. But that condition passes away as soon as its cause evaporates, which is usually in a few hours. Then, too, there may be diseased conditions of the brain which do not disturb the serenity and stability of the mind—that is, some minds are so strong that they hold themselves in proper poise even when the home of that mind (the brain) is in a disordered state.

From a medical standpoint, insanity means mental aberration due to a diseased condition of the brain. From a legal standpoint, insanity means mental unsoundness developed to such a degree that the victim is relieved from responsibility in case he should commit a crime. Or the mental disorder is carried to such an extent that the afflicted person cannot assume responsibility, or perform the ordinary duties of life, such as the making of a will, the conveying of property, the contracting of debts, or the incurrence of the solemn obligations of matrimony.

Thus you will see that insanity from a medical standpoint and insanity from a legal standpoint differ mainly in degree. A person suffering with simple melancholia might be considered insane and in need of medical treatment, while at the same time this person could exercise judgment, assume responsibility, and perform the ordinary duties of life. But when insanity has developed to such an extent that self-control is lost, or greatly impaired, and judgment and will are seriously disturbed, or reduced in action, then the person is insane from a legal standpoint.

A delusion is a false belief. There are both sane and insane delusions. A sane delusion is a false belief which comes as a result of imperfect education. A child may be taught to believe in Santa Claus, and he may actually put all his faith in that supposed individual. But this false belief in Santa Claus is a sane and harmless delusion. It is a delusion which the child outgrows when he gets a little further on in life. An insane delusion is a false belief independent of education or teaching, and it springs from a diseased condition of the brain. If a man becomes sleepless, restless, and expansive in his ideas by reason of an inflammatory condition of the brain, and while actually poor he comes to think of himself as worth a hundred millions of dollars, he is said to have an insane delusion.

We will now proceed to the consideration of delusions in their relations to positive insanity. These delusions are multitudinous in number, and of the most diverse and opposite character. They sweep the gamut of demoralized human passion. They fill the cup of their possessor with the gall of intensest sorrow, or they cause it to overflow with perpetual joy. They conjure up the gloomiest forebodings of future ills, or they arch the troubled sky of the desponding with a rainbow of ecstatic hope. They plunge their victim into deepest hell of despair, or they bear him aloft to some heavenly elysium. Such are the diverse emotions and pathways of those who are given over to the baleful influences of insane delusions.

Man's natural course is of an even tenor, and whatever produces undue exaltation or depression tends to the dethronement of human reason. A natural division of delusions may, therefore, be made under two heads,—namely, delusions made manifest by mental exaltation, and delusions which grow out of or are the effects of profound mental depression. In the former case incoherency of thought and constant change of ideas are quite common. In the latter a steady and fixed contemplation of a single idea is noticeable. In either case the cause of delusion rests in some abnormal condition of the brain. The most marked delusions are those of the general paretic, whose tendencies to ideas of grandeur and exhaustless wealth are well-known. In these cases there are changes in the membranes and cortex of the brain. Inflammatory adhesions are usually found upon the surfaces of the anterior and middle lobes of the brain in the paretic. In mania, where the delusions are remarkably kaleidoscopic in their manifestations, there is usually an inflammatory condition of the blood vessels themselves, which conditions, often varying, may account for the marvellous variations of mental action and the development of protean-hued delusions. In melancholia there is a greater fixedness of mental aberration than in mania, and there is also greater uniformity of pathological change, the usual condition of the brain in melancholia being that of passive venous congestion.

Delusions may result from a diseased condition of the brain, produced by either internal or external impressions. For instance, as a result of disease located primarily in the lungs, the heart, the liver, the stomach, the kidneys, or the bowels, the brain may be so impressed by reflex action that the victim comes to believe that he is on fire, that he is made of glass, that he has an animal in his abdomen, or that he is possessed by the devil. On the other hand, a person may receive an unpleasant impression from the sight of some horrible object, or from some action on the part of those around him, and such impression, developing an irritation of the brain, may come to produce at first a false conception of fact, and finally a delusion that he is being pursued, or poisoned, or injured, or robbed, or slandered. In the same way these impressions may stimulate the faculties of imagination and hope until the patient concludes that he is the possessor of boundless wealth, or holds sway undisputedly over the realms of imaginary empire.

An hallucination is "a sensation without an object," according to M. Ball of Paris. Thus it is said that an individual who hears voices when no sound strikes the ear has an hallucination. Hallucinations, to speak plainly, are false perceptions through any one of the senses. There are hallucinations of hearing, of sight, of smell, of taste, and of feeling.

Hallucinations are of two varieties: (1) Those which indicate a temporary and unimportant diseased condition of the brain, as, for instance, visions and nightmare, particularly in the young; and, (2) those which indicate profound mental aberration. As a result of a simple congestion, a person may see two objects on the wall where but one exists; or he may see stars or rings floating in the air, or angels in the sky. As the result of a drinking bout, a person may see snakes, or black dogs, or vermin. The same effects may be produced temporarily by such drugs as Belladonna, Stramonium, or Cannabis Indica.

Harmless hallucinations are temporary in their nature, and the victim may often be brought to realize their falsity. Hallucinations indicating insanity are fixed, permanent, and intractable in their nature. The insane man constantly reiterates what he supposes to be a fact, that he sees animals or objects, or that he hears voices, and no amount of argument or ocular demonstration will relieve his mind from the erroneous conclusions which he draws from these false perceptions. Sometimes a patient will temporarily deny that he is troubled with hallucinations, but this denial is generally of short duration.

Now it often happens that delusions spring up in the mind as a result of hallucinations. Hallucinations affect the sensory motor ganglia. Delusions find their home in the inhibitory motor centers, or centers held in check by the influence of other nerve centers. As in the ordinary action of the brain, we first receive impressions and then perceptions, and form conclusions and judgments by the transmission of these impressions from one set of brain cells to another, so among the insane these false perceptions make their impress upon the primary sensory ganglia, and finally transmit these impressions to the ideational centers. The natural result of these impressions is a false judgment of external things, and hence a false belief. And as a natural sequence of these false beliefs, we have that unnatural speech or action which indicates insanity, or a departure from the normal mental status of the individual.

It is generally considered among alienists that the presence of hallucinations in a case of insanity is an unfavourable symptom. The reason for this, we believe, lies in the fact that those portions of the brain which have been most thoroughly developed by constant use, and which are therefore the strongest, have become diseased. The ideational centers may remain dormant and inactive from lack of use, but those centers which receive impressions of external things through the senses are always, from the very nature of the things, subjected to steady and persistent toil; consequently they become hardened by use, like the brawn of the blacksmith, and are therefore enabled to resist the ordinary attacks of disease. Hence, when these strongholds of brain power are broken down by overuse, and their best forces are scattered by the blinding storm of insanity, their rebuilding becomes a matter of grave and protracted doubt.

Physically speaking, hallucinations are due to imperfect, or insufficient, or changed, or defective nutrition of the brain substance. They may arise from congestion, from anemia or from atheromatous condition of the vessels, which latter may produce an irregular blood supply.

"It is a singular fact," says Blandford, "that a person who is blind, either from disease of the external organ or the internal sensory ganglia, may yet see with the mind's eye, and reproduce in memory the appearance of objects which he has stowed away. Now we may suppose that in case of an hallucination, the internal organ is excited not from without, as ordinarily happens, but downwards from the ideational portion of the brain. Accustomed, however, as he is to connect all the sensations experienced with the external organ and the external world, the patient fails to perceive, sometimes at any rate, that the excitation is from within, and is firmly impressed with the belief that the sight, which the organ of sight apparently sees, and the voice he apparently hears, comes from without and not from within. The idea strikes his sensory ganglia so forcibly that the shadow becomes a reality, which perchance may not be removable by demonstration or argument." In the main, we think this idea of the learned doctor is correct. We have had under our charge several blind people, whose blindness was acquired. These have been insane, and have experienced hallucinations of sight. We have known deaf people to be troubled with hallucinations of hearing. But we have never known a person who was born blind or deaf to be afflicted with hallucinations of sight or hearing. It seems, therefore, necessary, in order that the ideational centers may produce a conception of external objects or sounds, that they shall first have been the recipients of similar conceptions through external impressions.

As we have already stated, persons suffering with hallucinations do not readily recover. We may state, however, that hallucinations of sight among those suffering from acute insanity do not preclude recovery. Hallucinations of hearing are considered more unfavorable than those of seeing. Even here, however, we may not pronounce an utterly unfavorable prognosis. Other conditions are to be considered in our final judgment of the case.

Hallucinations of taste are usually very persistent. One of our patients has for several years had an hallucination that her tongue is covered with ink or blood. Upon this symptom we gave an unfavorable prognosis, and time has too sadly proven the certainty and the validity of that opinion.

Hallucinations of feeling are, fortunately, quite uncommon. When once established, however, their victims rarely yield them up. One patient thinks that she is turning into bone; another that he has a child in his abdomen; another that her heart and lungs are being cut out; while still another feels kerosene trickling down the back, and thinks that somebody is setting fire to it. These are all hallucinations of feeling which breed fixed and permanent delusions.

An illusion is a mistaken perception. The victim may see a ball rolling on the floor, and may fancy that it is an animal coming to destroy him. A person may hear the sighing of the wind, and believe that he hears angels singing to him, or demons threatening him with some dire disorder. These are illusions. They partake somewhat of the character of hallucinations, but are still more closely allied to delusions. The latter is a false belief relating to some physical, or mental, or spiritual fact—that is, relating to some of the ordinary experiences or phenomena of life, —while the former also relate to some material existence whose qualities or attributes are mistaken by the beholder.

Like an hallucination, an illusion may be of temporary or transient nature; or, if prolonged, the patient may still be convinced of its falseness, in which case these spectral sights produce no marked change in the conduct or habits of thought of the individual. It is a blessed fact that visions strange may rise up before us, yet fail to frighten us from the path of sanity; and it is also a consoling truth that "thoughts impure may pass through minds of angels and of men, and leave no stain". In the case of man, this results because the brain is healthy. It is only when the hot iron of disease has seared and scorched the brain to its depths, that the mind is distorted in all its workings; and it is then only that delusions, and hallucinations, and illusions creep like shadowy ghosts into the dilapidated and ruined chambers of the soul, and refuse to be exorcised by the wand of modern science.

Mental unsoundness is designated by several terms. The victims of this unsoundness are called insane; they are called lunatics because it was once supposed that the moon affected the insane; they are called crazy because the term signifies an unnatural degree of mental excitement. When speaking of the insane in their presence, you should never use any of these old-fashioned terms, but you should speak of them as mental invalids, suffering with distresses of the mind. Such persons demand as much tender care and kindly sympathy as do those who suffer with physical pain.

Requirements for Legal Commitment

The requirements for a legal commitment to a hospital for the insane in the State of New York are as follows:

HISTORY AND CLASSIFICATION OF INSANITY

*"A person alleged to be insane, and who is not in confinement on a criminal charge, may be committed to and confined in an institution for the custody and treatment of the insane upon an order made by a judge of a court of record of the city or county, or a justice of the supreme court of the judicial district, in which the alleged insane person resides or may be, adjudging such person to be insane, upon a certificate of lunacy, made by two qualified medical examiners in lunacy, accompanied by a verified petition therefor, or upon such certificate and petition, and after a hearing to determine such question, as provided in this article. The commission shall prescribe and furnish blanks for such certificates and petitions, which shall be made only upon such blanks. An insane person shall be committed only to a state hospital, a duly licensed institution for the insane, or the Matteawan State Hospital, or to the care and custody of a relative or committee, as hereinafter provided. No idiot shall be committed to or confined in a state hospital. But any epileptic or feeble-minded person becoming insane may be committed as an insane person to a state hospital for custody and treatment therein.

"The certificate of lunacy must show that such person is insane and must be made by two reputable physicians, graduates of an incorporated medical college, who have been in the actual practice of their profession at least three years, and have filed with the commissioner a certified copy of the certificate of a judge of a court of record, showing such qualifications in accordance with forms prescribed by the commission.

"Such physicians shall jointly make a final examination of the person alleged to be insane within ten days next before the granting of order. The date of the certificate

* Chap. 545, Laws of 1896, Art. 3, sections 60, 61, 62, 63, and 64.

of lunacy shall be the date of such joint examination. Such certificate of lunacy shall be in the form prescribed by the commission, and shall contain the facts and circumstances upon which the judgment of the physicians is based, and show that the condition of the person examined is such as to require care and treatment in an institution for the care, custody and treatment of the insane.

"Neither of such physicians shall be a relative of the person applying for the order or of the person alleged to be insane, or a manager, superintendent, proprietor, officer, stockholder, or have any pecuniary interest, directly or indirectly, or be an attending physician in the institution to which it is proposed to commit such person.

"Any person with whom an alleged insane person may reside or at whose house he may be, or the father or mother, husband or wife, brother or sister, or the child of any such peson, and any overseer of the poor of the town, and superintendent of the poor of the county in which any such person may be, may apply for such order, by presenting a verified petition containing a statement of the facts upon which the allegation of insanity is based, and because of which the application for the order is made. Such petition shall be accompanied by the certificate of lunacy of the medical examiners, as prescribed in the preceding section. Notice of such application shall be served personally, at least one day before making such application, upon the person alleged to be insane, and if made by an overseer or superintendent of the poor, also upon the husband or wife, father or mother or next of kin of such alleged insane person, if there be any such known to be residing within the county, and, if not, upon the person with whom such alleged insane person may reside, or at whose house he may be. The judge to whom the application is to be made may dispense with such personal service, or may direct substituted service to be made upon some person to be designated by him. He shall state in a certificate to be attached to the petition his reason for dispensing with personal service of such notice, and if substituted service is directed the name of the person to be served therewith.

"The judge to whom such application is made may, if no demand is made for a hearing in behalf of the alleged insane person, proceed forthwith to determine the question of insanity, and if satisfied that the alleged insane person is insane may immediately issue an order for the commitment of such person to an institution for the custody and treatment of the insane. If, however, it appears that such insane person is harmless and his relatives or a committee of his person are willing and able to properly care for him, at some place other than such institution, upon their written consent the judge may order that he be placed in the care and custody of such relatives or such committee. Such judge may, in his discretion, require other proofs in addition to the petition and certificate of the medical examiners.

"Upon the demand of any relative or near friend in behalf of such alleged insane person, the judge shall, or he may upon his own motion, issue an order directing the hearing of such application before him at a time not more than five days from the date of such order, which shall be served upon the parties interested in the application and upon such other persons as the judge, in his discretion, may name. Upon such day, or upon such other day, to which the proceeding shall be regularly adjourned, he shall hear the testimony introduced by the parties and examine the alleged insane person if deemed advisable, in or out of court, and render a decision in writing as to such a person's insanity. If it be determined that such person is insane, the judge shall forthwith issue his order committing him to an institution for the custody and treatment of the insane, or make such other order as is provided in this section. If such judge cannot hear the application he may, in his order directing the hearing, name some referee, who shall hear the testimony, and report the same forthwith, with his opinion thereon, to such judge, who shall, if satisfied with such report, render his decision accordingly. If the commitment be made to a state hospital, the order shall be accompanied by a written statement of the judge as to the financial condition of the insane person and of the persons legally liable for his maintenance as far as can be ascertained. The superintendent of such state hospital shall be immediately notified of such commitment, and he shall, at once, make provisions for the transfer of such insane person to such hospital.

"The petition of the applicant, the certificate in lunacy of the medical examiners, the order directing a further hearing as provided in this section, if one be issued, and the decision of the judge or referee, and the order of commitment shall be presented at the time of the commitment to the superintendent or person in charge of the institution to which the insane person is committed, and verbatim copies shall be forwarded by such superintendent or person in charge and filed in the office of the state commission in lunacy. The relative, or committee, to whose care and custody any insane person is committed, shall forthwith file the petition, certificate, and order, in the office of the clerk of the county where such order is made, and transmit a certified copy of such papers to the commission in lunacy, and procure and retain another such certified copy.

"The superintendent or person in charge of any institution for the care and treatment of the insane may refuse to receive any person upon any such order, if the papers required to be presented shall not comply with the provisions of this section, or if, in his judgment, such person is not insane within the meaning of this statute, or, if received, such person may be discharged by the commission. No person shall be admitted to any such institution under such order after the expiration of five days from and inclusive of the date thereof.

"If a person ordered to be committed, pursuant to this chapter, or any friend in his behalf, is dissatisfied with the final order of a judge or justice committing him, he may, within ten days after the making of such order, appeal therefrom to a justice of the supreme court other than the justice making the order, who shall cause a jury to be summoned as in case of proceedings for the appointement of a committee for an insane person, and shall try the question of such insanity in the same manner as in proceedings for the appointment of a committee. Before such appeal shall be heard, such person shall make a deposit or give a bond, to be approved by a justice of the supreme court, for the payment of the costs of the appeal, if the order of commitment is sustained. If the verdict of the jury be that such person is insane, the justice shall certify that fact and make an order of commitment as upon the original hearing. Such order shall be presented, at the time of the commitment of such insane person, to the superintendent or person in charge of the institution to which the insane person is committed, and a copy thereof shall be forwarded to the commission by such superintendent or person in charge and filed in the office thereof. Proceedings under the order shall not be stayed pending an appeal therefrom, except upon an order of a justice of the supreme court, and made upon a notice, and after a hearing with provisions made therein for such temporary care and treatment of the alleged insane person as may be deemed necessary.

"If a judge shall refuse to grant an application for an order of commitment of an insane person, proved to be dangerous to himself or others, if at large, he shall state his reasons for such refusal in writing, and any person aggrieved thereby may appeal therefrom in the same manner and under like conditions as from an order of commitment.

"The costs necessarily incurred in determining the question of the insanity of a poor or indigent person and in securing his admission into a state hospital, and the expense of providing proper clothing for such person, in accordance with the rules and regulations adopted by the commission, shall be a charge upon the town, city or county securing the commitment. Such costs shall include the fees allowed by the judge or justice ordering the commitment to the medical examiners. If the person sought to be committed is not a poor or indigent person, the costs of the proceedings to determine his insanity and to secure his commitment, as provided in this article, shall be a charge upon his estate, or shall be paid by the persons legally liable for his maintenance. If in such proceedings, the alleged insane person is determined not to be insane, the judge or justice may, in his discretion, charge the costs of the proceedings to the person making the application for an order of commitment, and judgment may be entered for the amount thereof and enforced by execution against such person."

We see from the foregoing that in order to effect a legal commitment, the following requirements of law must be complied with:

1. A petition.
2. Personal service.

3. Examination by two qualified medical examiners in lunacy.

4. Judicial order of commitment by a judge of a court of record.

5. Statement of financial condition of patient.

Blank forms of commitment, together with initial history blanks, are furnished by the hospital when so desired and deemed necessary.

All town, county or city authorities before sending a patient to a hospital must see that said patient is in a state of bodily cleanliness, and provided with new clothing throughout, including shoes and hat. Between the months of November and April, both inclusive, there shall be provided, in additition to the foregoing, a suitable overcoat for male patients and a suitable shawl or cloak for female patients; also gloves or mittens.

I have given you the method of commitment. A very important question may arise in your practice as to whether or not a given insane person should be sent to a hospital. The rule you should adopt is this: You should send to a hospital, in the early stages of his disease, an insane person who is dangerous to himself or others. That is, you should send a person to a hospital who is likely to commit suicide or homicide, or who might, under the influence of his insanity, destroy valuable property, or endanger or greatly distress others by his excitement, and his unnatural speech or action. You should send acute or curable cases to a hospital for treatment when it is quite certain that the patient's chances for recovery are improved by such procedure.

You should refrain from sending persons to a hospital for the insane:

1. When the patients are very old and feeble, and cannot do much damage at home.

2. When the patients are young or middle-aged, but so very weak that their lives would be endangered by transportation from their homes to the hospital. Such cases should be kept at home until they are sufficiently strong to endure the fatigues of the journey. It sometimes happens that very weak persons are so excited by the journey to a hospital that they die soon after being admitted. A patient was brought to us after a journey of over two hundred and fifty miles, and he lived less than fifteen minutes after reaching the hospital.

3. Those who are not likely to be cured or benefited by treatment, and who are easily cared for at home. There are patients suffering from imbecility or dementia who can be readily cared for by their friends, and who, if sent to a hospital, would exert a depressing and injurious influence upon patients already received, and who may perhaps be restored to health.

Lecture V

MELANCHOLIA

We shall speak today of that form of insanity known as Melancholia. The term melancholia is from the Greek μελας, "black," and χολη, "bile." The name is founded upon the theory of a humoral pathology, the four humors, according to the ancients, being blood, phlegm, yellow bile, and black bile. Guislain gives as a synonym of melancholia the the term Phrenalgia, "brain pain"; Rush, Tristimania, "sand mania"; Esquirol, Lypemania, from λυπεω, "to make sad".

Melancholia is a disease characterized by great mental depression. It is an abnormality of mind to which all humanity is at times subject. It is a grim spectre of despair which enters every theatre of mental activity to molest and disturb. We meet it on the threshold of life, and through all our journeyings it hovers over us.

Some of the sons of men are melancholy by nature. They have bilious temperaments; they look upon the sunniest experiences of life through green and yellow goggles, and if such men make a feeble effort to escape from the spirit of melancholy she seizes upon them with renewed vigor, and in reply to all pleadings for freedom and happiness she echoes in their ears the cry of Poe's Raven—"nevermore".

"Melancholia," says Maudsley, "is a deep painful feeling of profound depression and misery—a great mental suffering. The patient's feelings of external objects and events are perverted, so that he complains of being strangely and unnaturally changed. Impressions which should rightly be agreeable or only indifferent are felt as painful. Friends and relatives are regarded with sorrow or aversion, and their attentions with suspicions. He feels himself entirely isolated, and can take no interest in his affairs, and either shuns society and seeks solitude, lying in bed, unwilling to exert himself, or he utters his agony in sounds ranging from the moan of dull ache to the shrill cry of anguish, or in ceaseless gestures of misery, or even in some convulsive act of desperate violence."

Causes

The causes which impel the inception and onset of this dread disorder are almost as numerous as the experiences of life. Still we may name among the prominent causes of melancholia the following:

1. Predisposition.
2. Physical disease.
3. Dissipation.
4. Work and worry.
5. Shock from sudden loss of friends or fortune.
6. Brooding.
7. Disorders of faith.

Predisposition.—Predisposition is an unnatural, inborn, inherited tendency to look upon the dark side of life; to make the worst of everything; to conjure up horrors that may never exist; to cross bridges before they are reached; to imagine that an enemy lurks behind every tree and stone, and that even tried and true friends are not always to be trusted.

Physical Disease.—One of the most common exciting causes of insanity is physical disease at or after the period of maturity. Whatever tends to deplete and exhaust the physical system tends to the production of insanity. Physical disease is produced by various influences, but chiefly by the reckless extravagance of the young in making undue drafts, either by toil or pleasure, upon the natural resources of the system. To be rich, to be great, to be honored, and to be loved are ambitions which fill the American heart. And the overzealous struggle for these prizes tends to the production of those physical diseases which culminate in insanity.

It frequently happens that the victims of long-continued physical disease become depressed. This may be the result of pain, or weakness, or exhaustion, or a feeling of helplessness, and loss of usefulness. The disease known as the grip especially exhausts the nervous system, and causes profound mental depression. Again, those who suffer with non-limited diseases are apt to formulate the idea that they will never recover, and thus they become depressed. It is well to remember, likewise, that a healthy person may experience a shock upon his nervous system through losses of some kind, and then become the victim of physical disease. At any rate, you generally find that patients suffering with melancholia are weaker than when in health, and that all the functions of the body are sluggish in their action. The bowels are constipated, the kidneys are inactive, the respiration is labored and incomplete, and the heart's action is apt to be slow. The blood is imperfectly purified, and a general venous stagnation ensues. The skin becomes dry, and greatly impaired in function. The bile is not properly eliminated. Coupled with this physical inactivity, we find, most naturally, a slow and painful working of the mind itself as a result of physical disease.

Dissipation.—By this we mean that excessive drinking, or excessive eating, or excessive exhaustion of the sexual system, either by natural or unnatural means, not infrequently results in a culminating attack of melancholia. At the end of a long drunken debauch, a man often feels such compunctions of conscience that he is driven into an attack of suicidal melancholia. Hence you read of numerous cases where a drunken spree is ended by self-shooting, or hanging, or poisoning.

Work and Worry.—Who can calculate the dangers that spring from the overwear of work and worry? No people in the world work harder than do the American people. This excess of toil might be endured with safety were it not for the added grind upon the vital forces of a worrying spirit. We toil all day for the accomplishment of a certain purpose, and worry all night, with fear and trembling lest the results of our toil may not be the ripest and the rarest of all possible fruits. The young worry about their studies in school; they worry about their appearance and their prospects when associating with others; they worry lest they shall fail to get rich; they worry lest they shall lose some strongly inviting prize in life. A great many women are timid and anxious and fearful, and look into the future constantly with strained and tearful eyes. They see lions in every path, and they worry lest they shall fall into their clutches, and come to harm. Nine-tenths of all the worry in this life is not only useless, but injurious; and nothing more certainly leads to a continued mental depression than worrying about the future of this or the next life.

Worry about one's prospects, and means, and acquirements is like sand poured into the bearings of a rapidly revolving wheel. The friction and the wear are intense; the bearings become overheated, and necessity compels oftentimes a dead halt, a cleaning out of the bearings, the introduction of the oil of rest until the heat subsides; and only after long and vexatious delays may any renewed attempts at progress be made. And sometimes worry so effectually destroys the bearings in the human vehicle as to preclude the possibility of repair, and the possibility of future progress. (If you would become philosophical and happy, read Menticulture by Horace Fletcher.)

Shock.—When a person suddenly hears unfavorable news, such as the sudden death of a husband, or a father, or a brother, who is absent, or when a mother loses her child after a brief illness, or when the breadwinner of the family loses his fortune through speculation, or his position through wrong-doing, or his health through recklessness of living, then comes a sudden and forcible impression which diffuses itself throughout and prostrates the entire nervous system. This impression, which causes the heart to momentarily stand still, and which nearly paralyzes the brain, is termed 'shock". The condition of the nervous system resulting from shock is recovered from only with great difficulty. The physical functions are so much impaired that they work only by a terrific strain of the system. The condition is like that of delicate machinery which has been hammered, and bent, and deprived of necessary oil to relieve the friction. Under the influence of shock upon the physical system, the mental state becomes one of depression and despair.

Brooding.—We have spoken of brooding as another cause of melancholia. Brooding differs from anxiety and worry in this: The person who broods over disappointment in life or ambition quietly seeks to keep his trouble to himself, while the victim of anxiety and worry is quite apt to give expression to his feelings, and thus relieve the strain upon him to a considerable extent. Quiet brooding over the past constitutes a most dangerous tendency to melancholia.

Disorders of Faith.—These are numerous and distressing. They tend to the formation of strange and wonderful delusions relative to the individual relationship between himself and his fellows, between himself and the great Creator above us, and between himself in his mortal sphere, and his relations to the undiscovered future. Predisposition, physical causes, overwork, worry, shock and brooding, are causes associated with daily life and present experiences. The disorders of faith are associated with those intangible subjects concerning present and future existence, concerning the mortal and immortal, concerning Creator, creation, and created. It would be well if those who suffer from disorders of faith could cultivate a better philosophy, and restrain their unfettered imaginings, and like little boys before they learn to swim, they should only paddle near the shores of time.

Forms

Melancholia may be divided as follows:
1. Simple melancholia.
2. Acute melancholia.
3. Subacute melancholia.
4. Chronic melancholia.
5. Melancholia with stupor.
6. Melancholia with agitation.
7. Melancholia with resistance.
8. Acute delirious melancholia.
9. Hypochondriacal melancholia.

Symptoms, Courses, and Cases

Simple Melancholia.—This form of insanity is characterized by a continued depression without the formation of concrete delusions. An attack of the "blues" is the mildest type of simple melancholia. Beyond this, you will find those who are suffering with continued strain of losses, and without experiencing any especial shock or sudden attack, they pass gradually into a fixed state of simple melancholia. This state sometimes leads to a more severe form, but until new developments arise the victim of simple melancholia thinks that he is only "bilious".

A strange feature of simple melancholia is that the patient oftentimes can give no reason for the change that has "come o'er him like a summer's cloud". In the language of Shakespeare, he may say to himself: "I have of late (but wherefore I know not) lost all my mirth, foregone all custom of exercises; and, indeed, it goes so heavily with my disposition, that this goodly frame, the earth, seems to me a sterile promontory; this most excellent canopy, the air, look you, this brave o'erhanging firmament, this majestic roof fretted with golden fire, why it appears no other thing to me than a foul and pestilent congregation of vapors."

Acute Melancholia.—Acute melancholia is generally the result of some sudden mental shock produced either by loss of friends, reverse of fortune, desertion or seduction, physical disease or pain, or by any of the great overwhelming casualties, or calamities, or convictions of life. At first a sudden shock of grief or despair from remorse may merely darken or cloud the life of its victim. Then come misconceptions of the mission and ends of life. Customary occupations and pleasures are forsaken; the natural secretions and excretions of the body are hindered and impeded. As the courage fails, so likewise the strength. The patient loses his appetite, and as nourishment is taken in insufficient quantities, and but poorly assimilated, the patient wastes in flesh, and becomes wrinkled and prematurely aged in appearance.

The person suffering from acute melancholia generally looks down; keeps quiet; scowls; refrains from talking; dislikes to be spoken to; is averse to the consolations of friends; and in many ways he presents outwardly those appearances of degeneration which are characteristic of inward hopelessness.

At first the victim of acute melancholia may seem to have no definite delusion, but after a short time the vast and formless feelings of profound misery take shape as a concrete idea. In other words, his sorrow is condensed and crystallized into some definite delusion. The patient comes to believe that he has committed a great crime, for which he must suffer death; that he has blasted the happiness of his family; that he is possessed of the devil, or that he is the victim of a persistent and cruel persecution by electricity, or by magnetism. And again, he has committed the unpardonable sin, and is forever damned. The delusion is not the cause of the feeling of misery, but is engendered by it. These unhallowed fancies take shapes according to the patient's culture and education. What the uneducated and superstitious attribute to witches or to devils the man of culture ascribes to electricity, or magnetism, or political conspiracy. In certain cases it is striking how disproportionate the delusion is to the extreme mental anguish; how inadequate it is as the expression of it. One whose agony is that of the damned will swear that it is because he has drunk a glass of beer which he should not have done, or because he has muttered a curse when he ought to have offered a prayer. With him who believes that he is doomed to infinite and eternal misery, it is not the delusion but the affective disorder that is the fundamental fact. There can be no adequate or definite idea of the infinite or eternal, and the insane delusion of eternal damnation is but the vague and futile attempt at expressing an unutterable real suffering.

It is noteworthy, again, how much the affliction of the melancholiac subsides when a definite delusion is established.

The vast feeling of vague misery which possessed the whole mind has undergone systematization in definite morbid actions. When the delusion is not active, but reposes in the background, the patient may be tolerably cheerful.

A suicidal feeling is common in cases of acute melancholia. Hence a patient suffering with this form of insanity should always be watched and cared for, lest in some paroxysm of agony he should seek both to kill some of his friends and himself.

Acute melancholia may terminate in recovery, or it may culminate in an attack of mania. If death ensues, it usually results from exhaustion.

No 5,414, æt. 28, unmarried, was a case of acute melancholia in a woman, resulting from overwork, and a love affair of an improper nature. The patient was a dressmaker, hence her life was necessarily sedentary, and the opportunity for exercise in the open air was limited. Such conditions are apt to produce tendencies to mental depression. The duration of the attack previous to admission to the hospital was about six months. When she came under our care the patient's general health was much impaired, and she had lost considerably in weight. The mental condition was that of profound depression, coupled with anxiety, She was also suicidal, and had threatened to kill others. It is not uncommon for a case of suicidal melancholia to make an assault upon others just previous to self-killing. People who try to kill others, and then try to kill themselves, labor perhaps under the old-time theory that "misery likes company".

The patient in question was sleepless, emaciated, and showed numerous scars and abrasions from self-mutilation. She was also constipated, and had a poor appetite. The will power was very weak, and she needed constant reassurances from nurses and doctors to the effect that her "soul was *not* lost". The expression in her face was that of hopelessness, which is so characteristic of acute melancholia, and yet the patient was tractable, and willing to obey the directions of the attending physicians. In a short time, under suitable care, she was taking liquid food in abundance, and sleeping better than at first. She also became more cheerful in spirits. About six weeks after admission to the hospital, she was troubled with sexual excitement at times, and had difficulty in keeping her mind off improper subjects. She had amorous dreams. This revival of activity in the sexual organs is sometimes an indication of improvement in cases of melancholia. In due time the menstrual function was renewed, and there was an improvement in spirits, and an increase in flesh. Having commenced to improve, the gain in bodily weight and in lightness of spirits was steady, until she made a full recovery. She went home in less than six months from the date of her admission. Her weight was 127 pounds, showing a gain of 22 pounds during her stay in the hospital.

The remedies which this patient received while under treatment were Ignatia, Picric Acid, Pulsatilla, Cantharis, and Cimicifuga.

Here was a case of acute melancholia in a young person, caused by what seemed to her an overwhelming misfortune, and which brought on all those mental and bodily symptoms which make the diagnosis clear and positive. When placed under treatment, and compelled to live in a careful and methodical way, she became more philosophical and serene in mind. The gain in bodily weight was synchronous with the resumption of normal and elastic spirits. Every such case is an exemplification of the old adage, to the effect that a sound mind is to be found only in a sound body. The rebuilding of the physical health in a worn, emaciated and depressed individual, is the first step toward a satisfactory recovery.

Subacute Melancholia.—Under the head of subacute melancholia we class those cases which, from a natural predisposition, incline to a survey of life from the dark side. It is often difficult to determine in this class where sanity leaves off and insanity begins. The patients do not present the marked objective symptoms of mental agitation and physical decay which present themselves in acute melancholia, nor do they develop the fixed delusions so generally held by those suffering with the chronic form.

Subacute melancholiacs are mercurial in their nature, now rising to heights of sunny pleasure, and again slowly sinking to the depths of despondency. Such cases may recover, or they may drift into a chronic state. If they do recover, they are quite likely to suffer relapses. Their only hope is to join their fortunes with those who are strong, vigorous, and exuberant in spirits. They should live in the mountains, and in the open air.

Chronic Melancholia.—Chronic melancholia is the terminus of all other forms of spirit depression. It is the inevitable goal of continued mental shock, and worry, and brooding, and physical decay. The term is an epitome of all the disappointments of fickle fortune. The condition is a sarcasm upon human happiness, and the ultimate of vengeful fate. The means to this end are false and unsatisfying philosophies. Its field of operation is wide as the world, and the number of victims which this Giant Despair claims for his own is as myriad and legion.

Chronic melancholia is a grim and ghastly entity; a fetid reminder of better and brighter days; a sad relic of unprofitable and useless existence; a symbol of blasted hopes, broken plans, and a ruined life.

Patients suffering with chronic melancholia may live for years, mourning constantly over their fate, repeating daily their threadbare delusions; always looking into the darkness, and never seeing a ray of sunlight, until at last, worn and wasted by useless worriments and forebodings, their lives are finally exhausted, and their spirits shattered by continued beatings against the bars of relentless fate

Phthisis, marasmus, dropsy or death from exhaustion are the sequelæ of chronic melancholia, although occasionally a case recovers.

Just here we desire to present a brief history of a remarkable case. The case is remarkable in these particulars: First, from overwork and over-anxiety the patient passed into a condition of acute melancholia; secondly, from acute melancholia she passed into a condition of subacute mania, with marked delusions and semi-exaltation; thirdly, she subsided into the passive, non-elastic state which may be described as subacute melancholia; fourthly, she passed into chronic melancholia; and fifthly, after a lapse of ten years, she fully and substantially recovered.

Miss W., æt. 29, while overtaxed from constant daily labor as a teacher, was subjected to excessive mental excitement, agitation and anxiety from sympathy for a sister who was in great danger during instrumental labor. She was also much overworn by the subsequent illness and death of the sister's child, the care of which fell heavily upon her. As a result of these severe toils, she was attacked with headache, vertigo, ringing in the ears, and slight delirium. She had a rapid pulse, a flushed face, and wild, wandering eyes at times. Her tongue was coated white, and she had thirst, constipation, scanty urine, restlessness, agitation, and

MELANCHOLIA

sleeplessness. In about three weeks after the inception of her attack there was an apparent gradual amendment. The fever subsided, the tongue cleaned, the appetite and the general health improved, but there yet remained a disordered mind, more or less gastric disturbance, and some emaciation. She still remained restless and sleepless, and indulged in false beliefs and false judgments. The patient was strongly conceited, and had full faith in the correctness of her own judgments; fancied that her friends were all insane; that people were constantly watching her; was in dread of being buried alive; often fancied herself a dog, and indulged in numerous other false impressions. With these false beliefs and judgments she had such recklessness, and such disregard for the rules and usages of the family, that she not only interfered with the ordinary comfort of her friends, but excited grave apprehensions in the minds of those around her, lest she should do them or herself some bodily harm. This patient was naturally affable, amiable, of nervo-bilious-sanguine temperament, and of cultivated and refined tastes. At times she was quiet, and again very restless, and still altogether moody and irritable.

The patient, after admission to the hospital, at first complained of pain in the back and side of the head, ringing in the head, constriction and stiffness about the head and face, a parched feeling of the mouth; tongue felt as if burned on the sides and tip, bowels constipated, sensation of fulness after eating, a numbness of the body, depressed spirits. She said: "I don't see any use in living if I can't do any one any good." She was worse in the house, and about sunrise; later in the day and out-of-doors she felt somewhat better. The patient was always self-conceited, and at times quite emphatic in the expression of her disdain for others. She was given Platinum, and this remedy was continued for some time. Four months later her menses appeared for the first time, and after that she seemed a little better for a while. She thought she was "coming out of a cloud", and that she would feel better again. Then she thought that the steeple, which was being put upon one of the new buildings at the institution, was a gallows on which to hang her. Soon afterwards she realized that she had worked too hard, and that this was the cause of her suffering. The following year she settled into a dull, heavy, gloomy state. Her active delusions had in a measure subsided; and at times she brightened a little, and then would settle to the old plane of living and thinking. Two years later she began to be a trifle more sensitive. Passing from a subacute to a chronic stage she became more irritable and suspicious, and was inclined to write a good deal. Her letters were fretful and faultfinding reiterations of her troubles and her woes. Again, she passed into a state of slight exaltation. She played upon the piano for the patients at regular chapel services for a time, and then sent in a bill for one hundred thousand dollars, reckoning at twenty-five thousand dollars per year, and charging for four years, when she had been in the hospital but three years. Later the patient complained of frequent pains in her head, and had several attacks of nosebleed. She felt as if her head were coming off; had frequent dreams; had a cough, with greenish expectoration, and much rattling in the throat and chest. For these latter symptoms she received at one time Mercurius Iod., and at another time Antimonium Tart. The next year she had frequent attacks of diarrhœa, which came on in the night and towards morning, and these were relieved by Podophyllum. She was troubled with hoarseness, but no cough. She also had smooth, dark-red, non-vascular erysipelas on the extremities. She had bleeding hemorrhoids, with constipation, and severe lancinating pains running up the rectum. The remedies for that year were Podophyllum, Phosphorus, and Corrosive Mercury.

In the early part of the following year the patient ran down to seventy-nine and a half pounds in weight; complained of neuralgic pains in the head, face and jaws. During the latter part of the same year she began to gain in flesh, and continued to gain until she weighed eighty-five and a half pounds. She complained that people were laughing at her; was tyrannical in disposition, and troublesome on the ward among other patients; complained of pains in neck, shoulders and arms, with numbness in the latter at times. She also complained of sharp, cutting pains while urinating. This condition was relieved by Cantharis. She continued to gain in weight, but the following year she became dull and sleepy at times, and had dull pains over the eyes in the forehead; was somewhat feverish, and complained of her heart feeling as if it would stop. The patient had a severe attack of tonsillitis, and there was considerable swelling in the throat. Gelsemium, Belladonna, and Iodide of Mercury were her remedies for this year. Early in the next year she began to improve mentally; was able to write sensible letters, and did not appear to have any delusions. She was very anxious to go home; menstruated regularly, slept well, and had a fair appetite. Her weight at this time was one hundred and two pounds. She then had a brief depressed period, and indulged in a crying spell, for fear she would go crazy again. The depression was very brief. In a short time she was better and more cheerful. Lilium Tigrinum was the remedy administered to quiet her fears about going crazy. Five months later she was paroled for a month to visit her friends, and at the end of that time returned to the hospital voluntarily. She then talked sensibly and rationally in every particular, and her speech, conduct and self-control were consistent with perfect mental health. She was then discharged from the hospital as fully recovered, just ten years from the date of her admission. She has remained well since leaving the institution, and is now earning her living, as she did before coming to the hospital, by teaching music.

Melancholia with Stupor, or "Melancholia Attonita."—This is a somewhat rare disease, but intensely interesting from the fact that it is confounded with primary dementia, or at least it simulates a state of utter mental failure. Besides mental depression and mental obfuscation, there often exists in the patient thus afflicted a condition simulating typhoid fever. Here we have melancholia, dementia, and fever in a single case. At first the claw-hiding paw of unaccustomed sadness is laid gently upon the doomed sufferer, and it is only when the capture is assured that the stunning blow of dementia falls upon the stricken one, and the sullen fever begins its deadly course. In such cases we find, first, self-depreciation, coupled with the motionless fear of melancholia; and again, there is embarrassment of thought, an intellectual inertia, a slowness and incompleteness of ideational conception that belongs only to dementia. (M. Baillarger). Thus we have a combination of both melancholia and dementia, a unification so perfect and harmonious as to apparently preclude separation. Now in such a disease there is likely to arise difficulty in the line of making a diagnosis. In short, we must differentiate between the new combination (chemically considered) and its formative elements.

Melancholia with stupor may be differentiated from primary dementia, "first by the expression of the countenance, which in melancholia is contracted, and marked by an intense although an immovable expression; while in dementia, it is relaxed and expressionless. Secondly, in abstracted melancholy the patient resists being moved, sleeps badly, and often refuses food. In dementia, he complies with the wishes of the attendant, has a good appetite, and sleeps well. Thirdly, in abstracted melancholy the bodily functions are more seriously affected than in dementia. The body is emaciated, the complexion is sallow, the skin is dry and harsh, and secretions generally deranged; whereas in dementia the body often retains its plumpness and the secretions are little altered from a healthy standard. Fourthly, after recovery, the patient who has been affected with abstracted melancholy is found to have retained his consciousness through the whole period of his disease. When recovery takes place from primary dementia, the past is found to have left no traces in the memory." (Bucknill & Tuke). Thus we distinguish this multiple disease from one of its combining forms, *i.e.*, dementia.

From melancholia we distinguish it by the primary intensity of mental anguish,—too deep for utterance—and by the subsequent apathy, apparent loss of the powers of thought, and utter disinclination to all mental and physical action. In the ordinary forms of melancholia the patient is generally able to express himself clearly and cogently, although he may labour under the delusive idea that his soul is lost, or that in the body he is about to suffer the pangs of starvation.

Now in addition to the mental status already described as existing in melancholia with stupor, we find in some cases a pathological condition of the physical system simulating typhoid, which both complicates the disease and increases its already dangerous tendencies. We think that this fever is usually the result of personal neglect, the natural outgrowth of the profoundly beclouded mental state into which the patient has sunk. As a rule, the bowels become loaded with a large amount of undischarged fecal matter; and this, like any other irritative foreign substance, induces a slow inflammation of the intestinal tract, with a consequent rise of temperature, and an increased frequency of the pulse. Accompanying the fever we have an intensely dry and hot skin; a thick, moist and heavily coated, or dry and coated tongue; loss of appetite, with obstinate refusal of food, and a somewhat hurried respiration. While some of the symptoms, mental and physical, simulate typhoid, we do not have the exhaustive diarrhœa of the latter, nor such a rapid failure of the life forces as may occur in zymotic disease.

During the febrile state of melancholia with stupor, which sometimes continues for several weeks, the patient is, at times, restless and sleepless, tossing the limbs about, and lying with open eyes, yet in a dazed condition; or he appears to be dull and comatose, and is aroused with the greatest difficulty. As a rule, the patient pays no heed to the ordinary demands of nature. The urine is either retained, requiring persistent removal with a catheter, or it is frequently discharged in the bed, thus keeping the patient constantly in a wet and uncleanly condition. The bowels are also remarkably inactive, and will remain dormant for weeks unless their contents are brought away by the use of enemas.

In this strange disease all the machinery of life is thrown out of gear; the smoothness of its workings is impaired, and the *vis vitalis* is changed to a biolytic force, dangerous as dynamite, and whose only impulse is to tear down the citadel in which it is lodged. And yet it is a disease which may be successfully treated and cured. The patient must be artificially fed with a soft rubber catheter through the nose. The bowels must be emptied by suitable means, and the bladder must be cleared of its contents at regular intervals, that is, two or three times in twenty-four hours. Such remedies as Baptisia, Ignatia, and Bryonia may be administered with the liquid diet through the nasal tube.

Melancholia with stupor is, as we have stated, usually ushered in with simple depression of spirits. This may occur without previous mental derangement, or it may ensue in the course of an attack of mania. We have had patients brought to the hospital whose disorders were rapidly and fully developed at home under the pressure of some social or financial disaster, and again, we have had others who passed into this state after suffering with other forms of insanity for many months. In either case we have found melancholia to be the first sympton. This, however, is speedily followed by dementia, that pitfall which lies at the end of insanity's high-way, and which has been fitly termed "the grave of the human mind".

Melancholia with stupor may terminate by speedy recovery, by absolute dementia, or by death. If the patient gets well at all, recovery ordinarily occurs within a few weeks, or, at the most, within from two to six months from the date of inception. The recovery is often as sudden and unexpected as was the onset of the disease. The temperature subsides; the pulse becomes softer and less rapid; the sick one sleeps, and awakens to find the stone of sadness rolled from the heart, while the soul's recesses, once darkened by despair, are again radiant with newly received light.

Profound mental shock may be classed as the prime cause of melancholia with stupor. Such shocks are most commonly experienced by women who are young, of delicate fibre, highly sensitive, and extremely emotional in their natures. In such persons the play of passion is often of a tragic character, and the blighting of affection, the loss of a child, or the sudden wreck of a fortune is sometimes followed by a benumbing shock, in whose trail march the sad sequences we have already enumerated.

Where melancholic stupidity occurs in the course of insanity already established, it is difficult to state the positive cause, yet even here we believe it to be due to some suddenly depressing or exciting emotion. How far one's natural sensitiveness is retained, in the ordinary courses of insanity, it is difficult to state. Sometimes, however, it is greatly increased. With this hypersensitiveness, which we often find, it is not at all wonderful that having found no relief in the oft-repeated, long-continued wail of words, the patient should finally cease to speak, "strangle his language in his tears", give himself up to utter abstraction, and thus find at least temporary respite from his real or imaginary troubles. And if the woes of life are not thus crushed, the victim may yet hurry on to the Lethe of that dull forgetfulness which leaves both hope and care behind. The cause of this partial mental paralysis lies in the fact that every emotion of joy and hope has been chilled by the rude touch of heart-breaking disappointment. The mad world is filled with the dark clouds of despair, and the most exalted maniac is at times "wrapped in dismal thinkings", and given over to "thick-eyed musing and cursed melancholy". Between this primary depression and the succeeding stupor which simulates dementia, there is but a single step. The fever comes later, but is inevitable unless the patient's bodily functions are watched and attended to by his friends.

Melancholia with Agitation.—Over against melancholia with stupor we have melancholia with agitation, where the person walks, or stands, and wrings his hands, and pulls out the hair, and chews off the finger nails, and picks holes in the skin, and moans and groans, and deplores the fate of life. Patients suffering with agitated melancholia are often greatly distressed over religious matters, and such cases are sometimes termed "religious melancholia".

Melancholia with Resistance.—This is another distressing from of melancholia. Patients suffering with this disease resist every attention and care. They resist being washed; they resist having their hair combed; they resist all attempts at dressing or undressing; they turn away from their friends, and either curl themselves up, hiding their faces in their pillows, or they lie straight on their backs, and turn away from every one who approaches them. Cases of resistive melancholia will often emaciate very rapidly, because they refuse to accept proper nourishment. They also become very filthy, because they resist the calls of nature, and are opposed to every attempt on the part of the nurses to relieve the overloaded bowels and bladder.

Acute Delirious Melancholia.—This very rare form of melancholia has been reported by Charles Henry Mayhew in Vol. I., West Riding Reports. It is one of the most formidable diseases which the physician is liable to be called upon to treat. There exist, in the main, the physical conditions of typhoid, or of acute mania, but instead of that mental indifference usually found in severe fever, or the reckless exuberance of spirits often noticed in mania, there are anxiety, unrest, hopelessness and despair. When hope has flown, and corroding care supersedes that apathy which is really a conservative force in fever, then, indeed, is the heart sick, and life in the last degree jeopardized. It is, therefore, a most potent fact that "the vital energies are more imperilled in cases of delirium where there is mental depression than in those cases where there is mental exaltation". The disease, perhaps, depends upon a state of septicæmia, or upon some morbid poison in the blood, or a disturbance in its constitution. As far as I am aware, the blood has never been chemically examined in such cases, so that we have no information as to whether changes exist in its physical properties or composition. The symptoms, however, point to some toxic condition in the great nourishing and co-ordinating fluid, producing destructive effects throughout the system. The febrile condition, the general weakness and uneasiness which mark the outset of the disease; its sudden incursion and quick implication of all the secretions and excretions; the rapid and extreme expenditure of flesh and strength, and the tendency observed in some cases to multiple centers of inflammation or suppuration, are all compatible with a poisoned state of the blood, or the presence in it of effete or deleterious matter. That one should suffer the delirium of despair, under such conditions, is not surprising.

Some one has said that prognosis is materially affected in diseases generally by a careful consideration of the emotional state. On the one hand, we find those who are delirious and depressed; and on the other, hilarious and jolly. When a patient laughs and frolics, however noisy in language or outrageous in conduct, the prognosis may be favorable. It is said that gaiety indicates a reserve force which does not exist in cases of depression. Thus we see that different types of mental disorder correspond with different abnormal states, and thus signalize with nice precision the progress of pathological changes in the brain. It is always well to make an analysis of delirious ideas, and to differentiate those which tend to anguish, dejection and gloom, from those which are buoyed up with hope, exberance and joy. Unless you can speedily and abundantly nourish the emaciated victim of acute delirious melancholia, and unless you can change and stimulate the current of his thoughts, you will be likely to lose the case

Now for a case or two. Miss E. J. N., æt. 30. The certificate of commitment states: "She sits in her chair with her mouth wide open, her face fixed on vacancy, while the muscles of her face twitch spasmodically. Sometimes she tightly closes her teeth and lips, refusing to take food or drink, imagining that it is poisoned. She refuses to speak; sometime screams wildly, and is violent." We noticed that her hands were tightly clenched, and she resisted every attempt at moving her arms. At times she seemed to be intensely frightened at some imaginary object. On the day following her admission the patient was restless and uneasy; her hands were moist and constantly clenched; the skin was hot, pulse high, temperature about 100. On account of her obstinacy, her refusal to eat, and constant twitching of the extremities, we gave the patient Zincum. For several days she slept but little; was very weak; failed to pass water, or to have a movement from the bowels; did not respond to remedies; and was barely kept alive by the administration of beef tea and milk through a soft rubber nasal tube. Twelve days later the thermometer in the patient's axilla registered $106^{5}/_{10}$, the pulse about 146, and respiration 52 per minute. All indications were those of a speedy collapse. At this juncture we prescribed Baptisia, five drops of the mother tincture in half a glass of water, a teaspoonful every half hour. In the afternoon an enema was given for the relief of the constipation, and a considerable amount of feces was discharged. At 9:15 in the evening the temperature was $105^{8}/_{10}$, pulse 140, respiration 46, showing a slight change for the better. On the following morning the temperature was 104⁷/₁₀, pulse 120, respiration much less rapid, skin not so intensely hot as on the day previous. The patient's bowels were still much bloated and tympanitic. The temperature gradually decreased from 104 to 100⁴/₁₀, in four days. As improvement so happily succeeded its use, Baptisia was continued at lengthening intervals. Then the patient began to talk. In reply to a question, she said: 'I feel better, but I don't know what I am." During the remainder of the month the patient continued to gain steadily. This improvement continued during the next two months, until complete recovery was the result of her treatment.

The foregoing is a severe and typical case of melancholia with stupor. One of the best features of this class of cases is the fact that under careful treatment and good care a large proportion of them recover.

We now present a typical case of acute delirious melancholia, and, as you will observe, the results were quite the opposite from those contained in the treatment of a case of melancholia with stupor.

Mr. H. W. W., æt. 54, married, good habits. The causes of his insanity were given as hereditary tendency, business troubles and worry. His father was insane and committed suicide. The duration of insanity previously to admission was one week. While at breakfast one week before admission, Mr. W. suddenly threw up his hands and said, "I am lost, lost." He was persuaded not to go to work that day. The next day he stabbed himself about one and a half inches over the left nipple, and on the following morning jumped into the river, but was rescued. For several weeks previous to this attack he had been unable to sleep, and was troubled with dreams when he did sleep. When awake he seemed to have a horror of something. He thought that because his father was insane he would be, and this led to a belief that he would commit a terrible crime, for which his soul would be lost. The day after admission he wished to go home, as he thought that he had no means with which to pay his board. He had no hope, whatever, for himself, and was anxious to die. He became excited, noisy, irrational, and tried to injure himself by striking his head against the wall. He accused himself of forgery, of ruining people, and of misrepresenting. His pulse was 120; the skin was hot; he was intensely restless, and thought he was about to die. He was given Aconite in water. While taking the medicine from a tumbler, he bit out a piece and chewed some of the glass, but this he was persuaded to spit out. He continued sleepless and suicidal, yet he had a good appetite for several days. At times he would not speak, and on one occasion he stared into vacancy without winking for about four minutes by the watch. He afterwards became terribly excited; tried to bite himself; was restless, desperate, and determined in self-destruction. His tongue was dry, pupils moderately dilated, and his appetite began to fail. The patient tried so constantly to injure himself by kicking about, that he bruised his ankles and knees, and disfigured his arms. At times he would yell for considerable periods at the top of his voice. At length he began to perspire very freely, and his strength failed. When his hands were free he tried to tear out his eyes, consequently his hands were placed in padded mittens. By reason of his long-continued mental and physical excitement, he gradually became exhausted and drowsy. He said he was all tired out, and yet he slept but moderately. He began to experience difficulty in retaining food. His tongue was dry and coated; his face pale and cadaverous. He said that he had no pain, but was "so tired". This exhaustion continued until he died, just three weeks from the date of admission.

The temperature in this case was moderate, ranging from 98 to 101. The pulse was likewise moderate most of the time, ranging from 72 to 108, and only twice rising to 120. The mental agony and the physical excitement were absolutely intense, and wore out in a short space of time a naturally strong and healthy man. The vigor and intensity of his mental and physical action might be likened to that of a dog suffering with hydrophobia. Such cases are almost hopeless, and, with few exceptions, they rush themselves into the grave in a few days. There is little or no use in taking such patients to a hospital. The jar caused by riding in a car or carriage greatly aggravates their condition. They should be kept at home, closely watched, restrained in bed, carefully nourished, bathed frequently in hot alcohol and water, and the issue patiently awaited.

Hypochondriacal Melancholia.—Last in the list of definite melancholias, we may name hypochondriacal melancholia, or hypochondriasis. This is a form of mental disorder where all the thoughts and beliefs of the victim are centered upon himself. He has the worst liver, the biggest gall, the smallest heart, and the most inadequate lungs of any one in existence. Such cases are forever reiterating the belief that they have an incurable disease; that they are afflicted with cancer; that their bowels do not move; that the stomach is being filled with innumerable gallons of milk; that some animal is gnawing at their intestines; that the heart is failing to perform its functions; and some of them go so far as to think that they are "going crazy". Now it is probable that in many cases the hypochondriac is afflicted with some functional nerve disorder, which causes pain and uneasiness, and which gives rise to the exaggerated belief that there has been some wonderful organic change in the bodily tissues. Hypochondriacs should be carefully examined, and they should be favored and humored as much as possible.

The story is told of a woman who thought she had a frog in her stomach. Her physician finally concluded to cure her of this belief, and one day gave the patient an emetic, and while she was throwing up the contents of her stomach he quietly placed a live frog in the bowl which contained the *ejecta*. Upon seeing the frog, the woman was relieved of her delusion, but in a short time she said: "Doctor, there must be some young frogs in my stomach." The doctor picked up the frog which he had placed in the bowl, and looked at it, and said: "Madam, that is impossible, because this frog is a male." Then she gave up her delusion entirely.

So long as the delusion relates simply to a supposedly diseased condition of the body, there is a fair chance for recovery. But if the patient comes to believe that there is a ball of fire in the bowels, or that an animal is gnawing at the intestines, or that a nest of little devils is being hatched out in the womb, or that the heart and lungs are being cut out and dissected for the amusement of the doctors, the chances for recovery are very limited. If a person cherishes the delusion that he is poverty stricken, and that he and his family are coming to want, we regard the case as a hopeful one, particularly if the physical energies are only moderately exhausted from refusal to take food. Those who think they have committed a great crime, or the unpardonable sin, do not readily yield up their delusions.

Melancolia, at the outset, does not seem to involve the intellectual faculties. The victim may talk coherently and reason cogently upon all topics except with regard to his dark and deplorable beliefs. When patients recover from melancholia they are often much happier than they have ever been before. They seem to rise to the loftiest heights of exuberance and enjoy each day of existence, in happy contrast to those desolate periods when they were suffering most acutely with neuralgia of the soul.

Prevalence and Prevention

Melancholia is probably the most prevalent form of insanity known to history. Especially since the invasion of the grip, we have been burdened with numerous cases of mental depression. Almost every form of insanity is at times tinged with elements of mental depression. General paresis is frequently ushered in with an attack of melancholia. The same may be said of mania; while hopeless and helpless dements sometimes brighten a little, and then, feeling their own weakness, sink into the abyss of despondency on their way back to utter fatuity.

The prevention of disease is a grander and more beneficent achievement than the cure of the gravest malady. The surest prophylactic against melancholia is the leading of a regular, natural and healthful life, and the moderate and reasonable use of all good things with which the earth is so bountifully supplied, and which may be had by those who exercise a proper industry in attaining them. Excess of youthful pleasures is always followed by the retribution of subsequent despondency. But youthful pleasures were designed for wise and noble purposes, and should not be utterly avoided. A man who refuses all good things and becomes an ascetic is in just as much danger of drifting into "innocuous desuetude" as the glutton is liable to tumble into the pitfall of reckless extravagance. Those who pursue the even tenor of their way, and live according to the Latin suggestion, *in medias res*, may never scale the loftiest peak which ambition may point out, and neither shall they feel the pangs of utter disappointment when they fail to reach the topmist crag.

To prevent melancholia you should live patiently and regularly, yet withal earnestly, and with a constant cherishing of good motives and aims of life. Thus you may accomplish an excellent life-work. Your destined mission is thus fulfilled, and you will be able to smile at Fate, and under every vicissitude of life you may be able to say: "I have neither the scholar's melancholy, which is ambition; nor the musician's, which is fantastical; nor the courtier's, which is proud; nor the soldier's, which is ambitious; nor the lawyer's, which is politic; nor the lady's, which is nice; nor the lover's, which is all of these."

The treatment of melancholia will be considered in another lecture, in conjunction with the treatment of other forms of insanity.

PATHOLOGICAL STATES

The pathological lesions in melancholia are sometimes difficult to discover—that is, in their finer aspects In a general way it may be stated that a passive congestion of the cerebral sinuses is a common condition The congestion acts as a dam, and prevents the normal flow of nutritious blood through the cortex of the brain This congestion of the venous circulation produces pressure which, if unrelieved, leads to atrophy, or wasting of brain tissue In melancholia with excitement there is probably an active hyperemia of the brain—a condition similar to that existing in acute mania. If the melancholy patient is quiet, and indifferent to surroundings or the inception of nourishment, the brain may become anemic, and even edematous. The nerve cells being unused in a normal way are apt to waste in such a manner as to favour the hypertrophy of connective brain tissue. Unless the brain cells are used in an active and judicious manner they will certainly atrophy, and the spaces thus rendered vacant will be filled with useless material.

In studying the pathology of melancholia, you will often find diseased conditions of the abdominal viscera, and to such conditions may often be attributed much of the mental distress which has invaded the life of the individual thus afflicted. In the brain itself we often find but slight evidences of disease even where the patient has died in his unfortunate and depressed state. But even slight pathological developments in the brain will sometimes reveal the fact that its mental occupant was overborne in a most destructive way by forbidden and abhorrent forces, until it finally gave up the contest against the "slings and arrows of outrageous fortune".

The track of a vessel, as it disturbs the surface of the ocean, is speedily washed wawy. The casual observer sees upon the sunlit billows nothing to proclaim the fact that a steamship has ploughed through those obliterating waves. But the keen-eyed and long-experienced mariner discovers upon the tellatale waters, oil from the machinery, and ashes from the pit, and a bit of sable ribbon torn by the winds from a black flag, and he knows from these that a stranger and a pirate has passed that way. So the phantom bark of melancholia may sweep along the sinuses, and glide up and down the arterial courses, vexing the shores of the cerebral convolutions, yet leaving but little of track or trace by which its ravages may be noted or measured. Yet skilled investigators, profiting by repeated observations, are fast discovering, and marking out with faithful hands and by unmistakable signs, the course and the character of this unseen but deadly enemy of mental health.

Lecture VI

MANIA

The subject of today's lecture is Mania. The term mania, from the Greek μαινομαι, "I am furious", means a raving or furious madnes. It is used to express all forms of intellectual or emotional excitement where there are exaltations of the mental faculties, from distorted impressions and imperfect consciousness at the outest, on to disgruntled reasoning powers, dilapidated judgment, disordered will, delusions of innumerable types, and hallucinations of various kinds.

Incongruity and unnaturalness of thought, speech, and action are characteristics of mania; and through all the workings of a thus unbalanced mind there run a more or less constant series of impulses to works of fury and violence. Hence, the term mania, a most fitting word to convey the idea of a human mind given over to the demon of unrest. In a general way, Shakespeare stated the case correctly when he wrote: "He foams at the mouth, and by and by breaks out to savage violence."

The form of insanity which we shall attempt to describe is a favorite form, so to speak, of writers in both ancient and modern times. Shakespeare's King Lear is one of the best classical models of acute mania tending to senile dementia in an imperious yet despairing old monarch. We find likewise cases of insanity in the writings of Dickens, and Scott, and Charles Reade, and Captain Marryatt, and in many other works of fiction. In fact, throughout all literature, these abnormalities of human nature come to the front, and display themselves as fascinating fantastical in the solemn procession of real or fictitious life.

Causes

The causes of mania are put down in the books under such heads as loss of property, mental anxiety, overwork, ill-health, injury to the brain, sunstroke, and many other expressions which denote that the victim has experienced during his earthly sojourn some unfortunate disaster in mind, in body, or in estate.

The general causes of mania are much the same as those which produce melancholia. In the latter, however, the shock which produced the disorder works in such a way as to cause depression, while in mania the causes of mental injury tend to the production of irritation and of excitement. In dementia, the causes of insanity tend to bodily exhaustion and mental failure, while in general paresis the shock of disease comes after long and unwise contact with worry, wine, and women. Perhaps the temperament of the individual determines, to a large extent, the form of insanity which will crop out in a given case. In the production of artificial insanity by the use of stimulants, you will find that some men become depressed after drinking; others become hilarious, boisterous, noisy, and pugilistic; others sink into the fatuous and besotted state of dementia; and again, others simulate general paresis by the development of a general tremulousness, a tottering gait, a relaxed and unmanageable tongue, and a heightened imagination.

The physical causes may embrace every possible disease of the brain, from a primary congestion to a terminal lesion of the substance itself. In searching for the physical causes of mania, we must examine the head, the thorax, and the abdomen. Likewise we should consider the state of the sexual organs, for diseases of the uterus and ovaries, with irregular and suppressed menstruation, often accompany an attack of severe mania.

Mania often follows in the wake of general fevers, and their exhausting and irritating effects upon the nervous system must receive a proper consideration. Suppression of the normal excretions of the body may sometimes result in a maniacal attack. Long-continued ill health, together with worry, and anxiety, and perplexity, and apprehensions of various sorts, may tend to develop at first a general irritability, and afterwards an exaltation of the mental faculties that passes beyond the limits of ordinary self-control.

Insufficient sleep is one of the greatest dangers to mental health. The habit of getting up too early in the morning is generally the offspring of necessity. Those who are poor, and who are obliged to work hard for a living, must, as a rule, by compulsion rise early in the morning. By too early rising, I mean the getting up of these unfortunate victims of circumstance before the mental and physical forces are thoroughly recuperated from the exhaustions and trials of the day before. This danger of early rising comes not only to the farming classes, but likewise to those who labor in the mills, and factories, and stores of the cities. The gentleman of fortune and the unworrying tramp are usually free from the danger of getting up too early in the morning, and are comparatively free from the invasion of insanity. To avoid the danger of too early rising, the working classes should retire as early as possible in the evening, in order to devote at least hours to rest, and physical and mental refreshment. The trouble with many is that they sit up late for purposes of amusement or through the necessity for toil, and then get up in the morning before they are fully refreshed by sleep.

In a general way, we may state that mania may result from any unusual shock or strain upon the nervous system;

or it may come after any unusual mental excitement in business, in politics, or in religion.

Now, while we may easily recognise some of the exciting or stimulating causes of mania as affecting immediately the individual, I think we must go back of the presence of worldly misfortune, and trace the tendency to mental disorder through channels of hereditary influence. No one doubts the fact of resemblance in families of face and figure. How, then, can we doubt the fact of inborn tendencies to either mental steadiness or mental eccentricity? There are those whose natural bent is toward incoherency of thought and action. Infants are born every day whose inevitable goal is that of insanity. The toxic influence of wrong-living and wrong-thinking pervades their whole being while yet occupying a chaotic residence in their father's loins.

The primary and subtle causes of maniacal excitement should be carefully studied and understood by those who are to become physicians and teachers in the world at large. The physician's advice should be sought in every case of prospective marriage. By restraining those who are unqualified for the duties and responsibilities of propagating their kind, we might, after a time, improve the temper and quality of the human race. Correct methods of living should be learned from wise doctors, and thus the preparation in early life for future marital duties may be made.

Lack of brain poise, brain strength, and brain soundness at the outset, and lack of suitable mental culture subsequently, are, we believe, the most profound causes of this intellectual aberration known to the profession under the significant title of mania. These causes are but rarely recognized, and still more rarely acknowledged. How much easier it is to tell the mother that her daughter has become insane through some real or fancied slight put upon her affections, than it is to say: "Through your own carelessness and wrong-living your child was born with a badly constructed brain." How much more popular is that physician who declares that the young man has studied too hard or worked too much, than is the medical adviser who, seeking the real cause, plainly states that the brain of the victim was bent at the outset, and never straightened by judicious fostering in youth.

FORMS

The variety of insanity known as mania has numerous forms which we shall classify as follows:

1. General forms,—namely, acute, subacute (paranoia), and chronic.
2. Special forms,—namely, acute delirious, recurrent, periodic, and circular.
3. Peculiar forms named from supposed causation; to wit, traumatic, masturbatic, syphilitic, puerperal, hysterical, climacteric, tubercular, metastatic, and post febrile manias.
4. Disputed forms, such as monomania and moral mania.
5. There is also a class of manias which may be designated by some peculiar sin or crime, such as dipsomania, erotomania, nymphomania in women, satyriasis in men, kleptomania, pyromania, etc.

SYMPTOMS, COURSES AND CASES

We will now invite your attention to a consideration of the symptoms and courses of those manias classified under the head of "general". The others will, by their names, denote their tendencies, although we shall again refer to the most important of them.

Acute Mania.—Acute mania is usually preceded by a

period of mental depression. This depression is accompanied by a disposition to brood upon a single, all-absorbing topic. Dr. Johnson, the great English moralist, in his famous work entitled "Rasselas", has traced with a master-hand the slow, sinuous advances of mental derangement He says: "Some particular train of ideas fixes the attention; all other intellectual gratifications are rejected; the mind, in weariness or leisure, recurs constantly to the favorite conception, and feasts on the luscious falsehood, whenever she is offended with the bitterness of truth. By degrees the reign of fancy is confirmed; she grows first imperious, and in time despotic. Then fictions begin to operate as realities, false opinions fasten upon the mind, and life passes in dreams of rapture or of anguish."

Struggling against these ill-defined and misty influences, the patient feels painfully the slow gathering of an unseen storm. He becomes anxious and apprehensive, wakeful and haggard. A sense of intolerable unrest pervades his entire being; yet he may for a time be able to conceal these sensations from his most intimate friends by calling to his aid all the reserve forces of self-control. Gradually sleeplessness occurs, and the appetite becomes capricious and irregular. Dark gloomy thoughts pervade the mind even as damp vapors infest the valleys. Delusions which he cannot banish creep in. The victim thinks himself followed, and turns often to look at his pursuers. He imagines that his life-long friends are failing him. He begins to suspect that his food is being drugged; that the medicine which he may be taking for some bodily ill is potent poison; that he is being practiced upon by electricity; that the air is full of baleful odors. Charged with these false beliefs his mind becomes a pent-up volcano, ready to belch forth at the slightest provocation. The whole current of life thus becomes gradually changed.

The victim's daily toil becomes a burden. Social pleasures lose their fascination. The coming patient is given over to seclusion and brooding. The slightest cross to his wishes provokes him to fits of anger. The least anxiety induces an ebullition of rage. He neglects himself and becomes shabby in person. He ceases to care for his family, and is inclined both to jealousy and hatred of those who were formerly dearer than life. Finally the great upheaval comes. The bonds of propriety are suddenly snapped asunder. The patient yields himself up to his delusions, and is by them impelled to the commission of the seven deadly sins. No description is adequate to the practical reality. Honest men are transformed into demons, ready for any criminal act. Pure women become shameless, obscene, hideous. Mania is human nature unmasked and unrestrained. It is a condition which shows up in lurid light all the depths of total depravity. As mania develops in the patient, wild, incoherent, bubbling monstrosities of thought are begotten in the brain. These make their presence manifest by impelling the sick man to loquacious and unchecked babble. Incongruous as each remark may seem to its precedent, there yet runs a thread of continuity through the whole mass of illogical reasoning, just as a red thread runs through all the cordage of the British Navy. There is a certain fixedness of ideas in spite of irregular modes of expression. Each day brings a repetition of the same thought, but often with original rhetoric. Thus we observe truth in the classical statement that there is method in the madman's madness.

The physical condition in a case of acute mania simulates, somewhat, the middle course of typhoid fever, although there is less rapid failure of the life forces. Where the mania is long established, the appetite of the patient generally becomes good, and, in fact, oftentimes it is ravenous. By the consumption of large quantities of food the bodily strength is greatly conserved.

Mania is a disease where daily and nightly physical and mental restlessness may be expected. In typhoid fever while the patient is restless he is also prostrated, and can usually be kept in bed. The maniacal patient, in many instances, can be retained in a recumbent position only with considerable difficulty. Typhoid fever usually runs its course in about three or four weeks. In mania, the patient may continue in a state of profound excitement for many months. The skin is commonly hot and dry, with now and then a light, or sometimes a profuse perspiration. The tongue at the outset is somewhat coated with a yellow or yellowish-brown coating, and the breath is indescribably offensive.

If mania progresses with marked severity, the tongue becomes red at the top and edges, and in fact is often red throughout with a tendency to get parched and brown. The lips are frequently dark and cracked, and there may be sordes upon the teeth. The face is drawn and haggard; the lines of intelligence deepen; there is a scowl upon the forehead, and the eyes are wild and glaring. The pupils are generally dilated, though occasionally contracted; the pulse is somewhat quickened, and is hard and wiry. It feels harder than the pulse of ordinary fever. Occasionally the pulse feels like a writhing whip-cord under the fingers. This is due to the intensity of the heart's action, yet the temperature in such a case is but moderately elevated.

While the victims of mania often eat well, there are some cases where eating is neglected, and where the patient might starve through inattention. It is the duty, therefore, of the physician and the nurse to see that such patients are sufficiently fed. The bowels are frequently inactive. The feces become hard, and are discharged with difficulty. It is not always easy to get a case of mania to pay proper attention to the calls of nature. Thus tremendous constipations sometimes arise. They may be relieved by injections of warm oil. Ten or fifteen drops of the mother tincture of Hydrastis may be added to from four to six ounces of sweet oil, and that makes a satisfactory injection for a bad constipation. The urine in mania is high-colored, often scanty, and loaded with phosphates and urea.

The mania case is often dirty, lewd, and quarrelsome. Some patients will eat their feces, and drink their urine, or smear the body and the room with the same. Some seek constantly to breed turmoil about them. They grossly assault those who are endeavoring to care for them, and if restricted, will complain of their treatment. Maniacal patients frequently bury the hatchet of truth, and dig it up again only when their reason is restored

The course of acute mania ranges from one to six or more months. The length of time it may last depends upon many circumstances,—upon the age, sex, cause, period of incubation, number of previous attacks and other conditions. It is never safe to predict a time at which an attack of mania will terminate. The disease has no certain or probable course. If it is a first attack, and the victim is young and of good physique, with a tolerably healthy family history; and if the patient has elastic spirits, and is readily impressed by favourable influences, the prediction of recovery may be limited, with approximate accuracy, to from three to six months. But since most of these cases are burdened with complications, it is unsafe to make any positive prognosis.

The following is a typical case of acute mania, together with the results attained by treatment:

Mr. H. came to the hospital with a history of having been excited recently at some religious meetings, which, with suspected masturbation, was assigned as the cause of his attack. He was of effeminate appearance, single, thirty-five years of age, and considered a careful economical business man. Two weeks before coming here he became flighty; bought things he did not need; had the idea that he was Christ; that he could cure all ills, raise the dead, produce magical growth of plants, or do anything else that occurred to his mind. He talked incessantly of these and other things, and as his ideas flowed faster and faster, his tongue became unable to keep up, and his words ceased to bear any coherent meaning. He had hallucinations of sight and hearing, and conversed by means of his soul with people not present. For two and a half months he was restless, talkative and destructive. Only now and then could any of his remarks be interpreted into anything like reason, yet his conversation was influenced by what occurred about him. He was often twenty-four hours without sleep, and in spite of an abundant nourishing liquid diet his weight fell off. Toward the end of this period, short intervals of calm occurred from time to time, to be followed in a few moments or hours by a full return of the mania. Then he became quiet, unless spoken to, when his speech, after a few minutes, would become confused, and this is turn passed away with the progressing convalescence of his mind. Meanwhile his weight increased; his color improved; he took an interest in the life around him; his cleanly personal habits returned, and five months after his admission he left the institution a well man. His remedies were Belladonna, Avena Sativa, Cannabis Indica, Arsenicum, Hellebore, Stramonium, and Hyoscyamus.

Among singular cases of acute mania I may give the following.

A boy, eleven years of age, while passing through a forest

on his homeward way from school, perceived a wild-cat, and heard that animal's blood-curdling scream. He ran home in great terror. He rallied from the shock, only to pass into a state of exaltation amounting to acute mania. The child was committed to the Middletown State Homeopathic Hospital. Shortly afterward his two young sisters, aged eight and nine, who had witnessed his convulsive and maniacal outbursts, were similarly affected, experiencing attacks of acute mania, and were likewise committed to the hospital. All of the children quickly recovered. While they were in our charge it was necessary to keep them in separate building for a time, that they might not see one another, and thus suffer injurious excitement. When considerably improved, they could associate with one another without detriment.

Subacute Mania.—This is a mild but somewhat persistent form of mania. The patient does not suffer from those violent outbursts of passion, or long-continued paroxysms of excitement so characteristic of acute mania, but he cherishes the same physical and mental peculiarities. The subacute mania patient is cunning, self-poised, and deceitful; and will often induce in the mind of the unwary the conviction that he is not insane. When, however, you touch upon his chief hobby, he becomes aglow with suppressed excitement, which is most frequently manifested by a certain muscular tremor of the body, a hurriedness of speech, and an unsteadiness of the voice like a person laboring under the effects of but partially restrained passion. At the same time a glaring brightness of the eye is also apparent. Such cases often fancy that every man's hand is against them and hence are exceedingly jealous of their rights. These are the patients who are always threatening to sue the hospital for damages, who are constantly plotting to escape, or who seek liberty by means of the habeas corpus. They not infrequently deceive a jury of the laity by their shrewd deceptions and apparent lucidity and cogency of reasoning. These cases are generally cleanly, bright, apparently cheerful, and while retained in a hospital keep themselves under good self-control. But their deceitfulness, tyranny over friends, and unchecked impulses to wreak revenge for fancied slights when at large, call loudly for proper care, restraint and treatment.

Paranoia.—This term is derived from two Greek words, παρα, "beyond", and νοεω, "to know or to understand". It is a subacute form of mental excitement characterized by delusions of persecution and wrong. It is really a form of subacute mania. The delusions are fixed and systematized, and do not readily yield to any form of treatment. Paranoia is usually the outgrowth of a high grade of imbecility. Paranoiac patients come very near being wise, and some would be able to carry in their minds a little wisdom if they were not so horribly over-burdened with conceit.

"The delusions of the paranoiac may be reduced to two, giving rise to the two recognized forms of the disease, viz.:

1. Paranoia, with delusions of persecution,
2. Paranoia, with delusions of ambition or grandeur.

The latter has been subdivided into:

(*a*) Religious paranoia,
(*b*) Erotic paranoia,
(*c*) Jealous paranoia, etc.

Delusions of persecution and grandeur may be associated primarily, or the ambitious delusion may arise as a logical outcome and explanation of the delusion of persecution He believes he is persecuted, therefore he must be great; or he believes he is great, hence his persecutions. In either case his greatness is assured, and his supposed persecutions explained. His hallucinations do not by any means always confirm his belief in his greatness, but if not they usually add to his persecution. He hears vile names applied to him, people on the streets mock at him, the cough or sneeze of a passerby is a signal of his enemies, and means harm to him; therefore, he argues that he is a person of importance of whom others are envious, and whom self-interest impels to compass his suffering and death. If he lives in a monarchy some fancied resemblance to the reigning family leads him to believe that he is of royal blood, and thus an explanation is furnished which satisfactorily accounts for his persecutions, and at the same time flatters his egotism and self-love." (George Allen, M.D.)

If these patients begin to cherish delusions in early life, and cling to them systematically for years, they are not likely to recover. Sometimes if the delusions develop later in life, and the patients are favored with proper treatment at an early stage, they may get well, or get enough better to become quiet and useful citizens.

The following case from the hospital records is given as illustrative of paranoia:

A. V., a captain in the civil war, wounded in the leg at Gettysburg, while fighting desperately after most of his men had left the field, was born sixty-eight years ago in Germany. He is a man who always fully appreciated himself. He was wounded in trying to hold a position after he had been ordered to retire. His own opinions, activities and accomplishments have ever seemed to him of prime importance. In his younger days he was able to keep them in the background, but after years of secret brooding over what seemed slights and insults, his self-esteem became morbid and delusions of persecution developed. He considers himself the most learned man alive, and spends hours every day in committing his theories to manuscript. He is a believer in evolution, and declares that by finding a prototype of the female hymen in a Florida fish, he has supplied the cap-stone of proof; and this is only one of his many pseudo-scientific discoveries. Before being committed to a hospital for the insane he thought Mr. Cleveland, then president, stole his war record, and hid it in the White House, where he proposed to find it by a personal search; and he ascribes his confinement since then to continuous persecution in the hands of powerful politicians. Still hope never deserts him; such a man as he is cannot be downed; and when excited he regales his caretakers with promises of chains and tortures when his friends, whom he has summoned by his wireless telegraphy, shall come with avenging hands to the rescue. At ordinary times he is a quiet, gentlemanly old man, with a penchant for making himself believe that young lady employees are detained here involuntarily, and that he is a knight-errant whose mission is to effect their release. He refuses to take medicine, because he thinks he does not need any. The medicine which was presented to him he pronounces atropine, and he is carefully keeping it to prove a conspiracy to take his life by poison.

Chronic Mania.—Chronic mania is that form of insanity where the mental disorder has continued for a considerable length of time. The term chronic insanity, is a somewhat arbitrary term. The word "chronic" is derived from the Greek, χρονος, which means "time". Consequently when we speak of chronic insanity, we mean an insanity which has continued for some definite or indefinite period. Some writers claim that a case of insanity may properly be called chronic after the disease has continued for a period of two years. Others deem those patients chronic who have been insane more than one year. The distinction is an arbitrary one, and liable to excite discussion. For practical purposes, I think we may call cases of insanity chronic after the dis-

MANIA

order has continued steadily for a period of two years or more.

Chronic mania may terminate by running into dementia, by death, or occasionally by recovery. Dr. Rush says that "spontaneous recoveries now and then occur after the disease has continued eighteen or twenty years". (Aphorisms in Rush on Mental Diseases). Dr. Clouston, with regard to prognosis in mania, says: "Where there is exaltation, there is hope. We do not pronounce a case incurable for a long time; so long, in fact, as the morbid brain exaltation lasts, and dementia does not supervene. Concerning all cases of mania, so long as intellectual activity continues, and mental failure is not established, we should continue treatment with a view to recovery." Nearly all cases of mania may be classified as either acute, subacute, or chronic.

The delusions of the chronic insane, though cherished with tenacity, are generally modified or toned down from the acute or subacute form. Some of them are of a most curious nature. One of our patients cherishes the sincere belief that she is an "atom of dust", and ridicules herself for speaking, or eating, or performing any of the ordinary acts of life. Another claims that she has not been born, and says that her head is on fire. Still another can never get the words right, works herself into a frenzy over words which get "all mixed up", according to her delusion. This patient thinks at times that the letters of the alphabet are all turned into s's and z'z, and that it will take a life-time to get them straight again; yet she always talks correctly, answers questions promptly and clearly, and is finely educated. Another patient has for years persisted each day of her life that she "never stole Charlie Ross", and "never burned Chicago". Mrs. A. says she is "the Saviour and the Judge of the quick and the dead". Mrs. C. thinks she is fed with bread from heaven, and water from the rock. These are brought to her daily by birds with tinsel wings.

The insane man usually thinks that all things center in himself. He is the hub of the universe, and thinks and talks as if he were the only person worthy of consideration on earth. Many of the insane are egotistical. They do not fraternize well with one another. They rarely listen to the delusions of others, but prefer to consider and repeat their own.

Special Forms

Acute Delirious Mania.—Here we have an intensified form of acute mania accompanied by delirium, and terminating ordinarily in exhaustion and death. A diagnosis of this disease is not always easy, since many times it bears a striking similarity to acute mania. We may be guided, however, by the temperature, which is higher in acute delirious than in simple acute mania. The inception of this disease is generally sudden, and the outbursts of fury are severe and appalling. There are occasional remissions of excitement, but they are simply lulls in the storm, during which the tempestuous forces gather renewed strength. The disease is marked by two stages: First, excitement; and second, collapse. During the first period the face of the patient wears a peculiar expression which has been described as "a mixture of incredulity and maliciousness". The eyes are brilliant and glaring, and roll about with great mobility in their sockets. The mouth is filled with tenacious spittle; the lips and teeth are covered with sordes; the tongue is dry and generally coated brown, or it may be clean and bright red. The patient will often grind his teeth for hours in succession (also general paresis), and he frequently manifests a strong aversion to liquids. Sometimes when hurriedly taking a drink, he will bite a piece out of a heavy tumbler as if it were a cracker, and will chew up the glass as readily as a boy can eat a candy chip. The skin is dry and hot, and imparts a burning sensation to the hand. The patient keeps up an almost continual motion. Frequently the hands are kept moving in circles about the head. Hallucinations of light are commonly present, and the patient often addresses some imaginary individual. Constant and protracted sleeplessness almost always prevails.

The prognosis in this form of mania is generally unfavourable. In this respect the disease differs from both acute mania and typhoid fever. The stage of collapse comes suddenly, and is almost always very brief. Now and then a case recovers, but this occurs only when the disease is recognized at the outset, and when prompt measures for relief are adopted. The life forces must be conserved by judicious care, and easily digested nourishment, and the administration of carefully selected remedies.

Recurrent Mania.—In this form of mania the patient is very excitable for a time, and then appears to have a full remission of all symptoms of insanity. But the invasions of disease are repeated at intervals, varying in frequency from one month to two or more years. A case is on record (but not at this hospital) of a woman who recovered from recurrent mania forty-seven time, and who finally died during the forty-eighth attack.

Periodic Mania.—This is a subdivision of recurrent mania. It is named periodic from the fact that the outbursts of violence recur uniformly at stated periods, as every month, or every summer, or every winter, or in the case of some females at every menstrual flux.

Circular Mania.—Circular mania is a rhythmical alternation of mania with melancholia. Sometimes between the extremes of exaltation and depression, there is a period of complete remission or recovery. An interesting case of circular mania was long under my personal observation. The case was that of a lady patient at the hospital under my charge who for years lived in the following manner: For four weeks she would lie passively in bed, and no inducement whatever could arouse her to any physical or mental action. During this period she was much depressed in mind, would scarcely speak, answered questions only in monosyllables, and ate sparingly, but slept a good deal. At the end of each period of decuditus she would brighten up, have an improved appetite, become cheerful and talkative, and on the day following the completion of this month of rest she would leave her bed, dress and appear upon the hall the most loquacious of women, the most ceaseless in physical activity, and the most imperious in her numberless demands. At times she would become intensely excited, obstinate and mischievous. During the winter season she was much more inclined to violence than during the warm and pleasant summer months.

Peculiar Forms

Traumatic mania.—Among peculiar forms of mania we have the traumatic form. In the cases which have come under our observation, we have noticed that the leading characteristics are restlessness, incoherence, vivid hallucinations, mistaken identities, muscular weakness, heat in the head, and at times a besotted, half-drunken, dazed expression of the countenance. As to the pathological states in traumatic insanity, Dr. Skae holds that there is a chronic hyperemia of the brain and its membranes; while Dr. Blandford asserts that we have "to deal with a minute molecular change—a change which may be due to contusion of the gray matter, caused by a blow or a fall, and producing an alteration in nourishment and growth of the part, in blood supply, or in the nerves presiding over it".

Clouston states that he has seen about twelve cases of traumatic insanity in nine years; and concludes therefore that "accidents to the head do not loom largely in the production of the insanity of the world". J. Crichton Browne, on the other hand, suggests that brain injuries, inducing insanity, occur at all periods of life, from forceps deliveries to the accidents of old age. We believe that many of the brain injuries sustained during childhood are forgotten; and consequently when insanity occurs, this subtle and remote cause does not figure in the history of the case; and in old age these injuries are concealed by the pride of the victim. After a careful inquiry as to the general experience of numerous patients, we have come to the conclusion that many insanities properly date their inception from a blow upon the head, inflicted during the growing and tender, or later periods of life, and resulting in minute and long-continued pathological changes in the brain. Almost all cases of epileptic mania are aggravated by brain injuries which arise from the tendencies of the primary disease.

We present a case of mental disease produced by direct injury to the brain; and likewise a case whose recovery dates from an accidental but severe blow upon the head. Thus we have what may be called traumatic insanities. and traumatic recoveries.

The first case is number 2,207. Mr. W. E. S., æt. 18; occupation, laborer; education, common school; habits, temperate; no record of insanity in the family. When admitted the patient was in good physical condition, and his history declared that down to the date of his injury he had been a bright boy.

About six weeks previous to his admission to the hospital, Mr. S., while standing on the top of a ladder, twenty-six feet in length, picking apples from a tree, fell to the ground, striking on the back of his head. He was carried into the house unconscious, and remained so for several hours. He remained in bed only one day. From the time of his accident to the time of his admission, he is said to have spoken but two or three words. He could not speak when admitted, but during his entire illness he was able to comprehend questions written upon paper, and would answer these questions readily and rationally in writing. In his writings he stated that all spoken words sounded like noises to him, but had no meaning. He could hear a low tone of voice, but not a whisper. In writing answers to questions, he did so quickly, and showed a clear comprehension. He asked questions intelligently by writing, and said that he had a dull, steady pain from the base of the brain down the spine to the small of his back, and this pain was aggravated by any sudden jar. On examination, the spine from the first lumbar vertebra to the skull was found to be very sensitive to touch and pressure. He said that exercise did not tire him, and for several weeks he was allowed to do as he pleased. He spent much of his time out-of-doors playing with a large Newfoundland dog which was much attached to him, and which attended him when he came to the hospital.

Five days previous to his admission to the institution, this patient became much enraged at his mother who would not grant some request he made, and he flourished a long knife and tried to injure her. On being shut in a room he broke the door and was very violent. His friends then had him committed to the hospital under my charge. When admitted, his pupils were normal in size, and the reaction was natural. The tongue was clean and firm, with no muscular tremor;

the pulse was 78; the temperature 98.4°F. The patient weighed 150 pounds, and seemed generally in good physical state. He had a good appetite, slept well at night, stated in writing that the pain in his head had ceased, and he deported himself like a bright, good-natured, active boy. But he could not hear distinctly, and he could not speak at all, although apparently comprehending everything that was written and placed before him.

Here was a case of motor aphasia, or aphemia (can write but cannot speak), resulting from a blow upon the head, with occasional attacks of maniacal excitement; the excitement being displayed by restlessness and ebullitions of rage, without any ability to give articular utterance to his emotions or passions.

Although the patient had been allowed to walk about as much as he pleased for nearly six weeks, we concluded it would be better for him to remain quiet. Consequently we placed him in bed, and kept him there. The second day after admission he caught cold, and wrote on paper that his head hurt when he coughed. Four days later, about 9 A.M.—he wrote on a slip of paper, "headache", and gave it to the attendant. About 11 A.M. the pain in the head had increased and at 11 : 30 A.M. he was rocking backward and forward in bed with both hands pressed tightly against his head, one being over the forehead, the other over the occiput and upon the seat of injury. His face was flushed, pupils dilated, and the eyes deeply injected. While an assistant physician was noting these symptoms, the patient suddenly removed his hands from his head, looked up like a person awaking from sleep, gazed about the room in an imquiring manner, turned to the window, looked out for a moment, then suddenly turning to the doctor he said: "Where in the devil am I?" These were the first coherent words uttered since the injury. This patient's mind went back to its normal position with a snap, so to speak, just as a dislocated bone returns to its socket when it is set by a surgeon. On being asked if he did not know where he was, he said: "Not in the least. I know I was picking apples when the ladder broke and I fell, striking on the back of my head. Oh, how it hurt!" On being told that it was some weeks since the accident, and that he was in a hospital, he said: "Why, that was the eighth of October, what day of the month is it now?" On being told that it was the twenty-third of November, he replied: "Tomorrow will be Thanksgiving day; a lunatic asylum is a queer place to pass Thanksgiving Day." When told that he had not spoken before since coming to the hospital, he said: "I must have been good company." On questioning him he declared that he had no memory of anything that had taken place since his fall from the ladder. For six weeks, time had been a blank to him. After he began to talk, his headache lessened. He was kept quietly in bed, and given hot milk and beef tea every three hours. The headache and tenderness along the spine soon passed away, and no symptoms of brain or mind trouble returned. He remained at the hospital under observation for three months, when he went home in excellent physical and mental condition. While his memory was dislocated for six weeks, he could, after his recovery, remember distinctly all the previous experiences of his life, and all new experiences, but he could never recall any incident that occurred during the six weeks mentioned.

The second case is No. 356. Mr. J. A. H., 24 years of age; occupation, clerk; education, common school; no insanity in family. He was suffering with the seventh attack of mania. He had been insane (during his last attack) three or four weeks previous to his admission to the hospital at Middletown. He had been in other hospitals six times, and each hospital visit had lasted from three to eighteen months. On admission he was noisy and restless. The first night he did not sleep, but devoted his energies to tearing up his clothes. He admitted that he was addicted to masturbation.

The second day after admission Mr. H. was tearing his clothes, talking loudly, and eating soap whenever he had an opportunity. At three P.M. he tried to swing on a gas fixture in a wash-room, and turn a somersault through his hands; but as he swung his feet up to his hands, the gas fixture broke and he fell, striking his head and shoulders upon a tile floor. He got up, walked about, and talked for twenty minutes afterwards, when he became suddenly unconscious. His breathing was stertorous; his pulse 80 and very strong; his pupils appeared about normal in size. Soon after he became unconscious, the face grew purple in color, and the muscles of the right side of the mouth twitched; the pupils were insensible to light; the eyeballs insensible to touch, and there was diverging strabismus. At 4 : 30 P.M. the right pupil was more contracted than the left. At 6 P.M. the pupils were normal; the pulse 80. The patient was groaning, and he spoke confusedly of feeling badly in the left groin. At 9 : 15 P.M. the pulse was 72; the urine had been passed freely; the patient was very drowsy, with occasional muttering delirium. On the following day the pupils appeared normal; the pulse was 80; the urine and feces were voided with difficulty; the patient was able to talk, and complained of headache in the top of the head. He slept most of the time that day. The next day he seemed to have recovered very largely from the effects of the fall, and on the following day, three days after the injury, he talked and acted sensibly; and he continued to do so as long as he remained under our observation. He remained willingly at the hospital for about two months from the date of admission, when he was discharged as recovered. Three and a half years after he left the hospital, I met his family physician who told me that this patient had experienced no return of insanity, and the he was one of the most active and reliable business men in the town where he lived. I heard from this case again, ten years later, and he was still doing well.

Here was a case that suffered seven attacks of insanity in a period of nine years. His previous attacks had lasted from three to eighteen months each. The period of recovery ranged from six to twelve months. He was entering upon his seventh attack when he received the injury, and judging from the past, his insanity should extend over a period of from three to eighteen months. But this blow upon the head apparently caused a recovery in three days, and this recovery continued for at least ten years, and, so far as I know, it has continued during the past twenty-two years.

This case of recovery from insanity, by means of a blow upon the head, is exceedingly interesting, on account of both the suddenness and the permanence of the restoration to mental health.

Syphilitic Mania.—This form of insanity is acquired through indulgence with those who have the syphilitic taint. It often springs from coarse brain disease induced by syphilis.

Puerperal Mania.—Puerperal mania is simply acute mania associated with child-bearing. Its causes are indicated by its name. Sometimes insanity comes on during pregnancy and before childbirth. Again, it may occur within a few days after delivery; and once more, an attack may come on several months after delivery, and during the exhaustion of lactation.

This form of mania is caused by excitement or anxiety,

or by exhaustion from over-flooding, or from protracted pain, or from the wastes of nursing. And again, the patient may become exhausted from the loss of sleep in caring for the child. As you may meet such cases in your early general practice, we will give you an example case of puerperal mania which came under my notice:

Mrs. H. C. E., æt. 27, was confined six weeks before being brought to the hospital. Three days after confinement she was attacked with puerperal fever which lasted about one week. When the fever subsided she seemed well mentally. Two days afterwards, and twelve days after confinement, the patient began to show signs of insanity. She was excited most of the time; was obscene, religious, noisy, destructive, and sleepless by spells. For a short time she imagined herself wealthy, but she had no fixed or continued delusion. The day following her arrival at the hospital she was very noisy and destructive. She repeatedly declared: "I am under this flag; my ship is forty-five; I came here under false colors." She mistook those around her for persons she had known before; when food was taken to her she broke the dishes; was very violent, and seemed to have hallucinations of sight and hearing which frightened her. The patient was given Stramonium. After several days of excitement and incoherency she became more quiet and better-natured. Then she complained of pain in the head, through the temples, and over the top. Her pupils for sometime were considerably dilated. At first she cared little for food, but afterwards had an excellent appetite. Some weeks after admission she began to talk quite freely to imaginary people. She also heard voices, but what they said did not seem to disturb her, as she was good-natured and jolly. On account of her jolly delirium, her tendency to destructiveness, and particularly her inclination to remove all clothing, we gave Hyoscyamus, and this remedy seemed to have a favorable effect for a time. At length she began to menstruate, and had a profuse flow of bright red blood. During her menstruation she became more obstinate and pugilistic than usual. Her pupils were largely dilated. On account of her intense ugliness, and destructiveness, and the dilated pupils, and the flow of bright-red blood from the uterus, she received Belladonna. A little later the patient was not only wild, noisy and destructive, and inclined to remove all clothing, but she began to smear herself and her room with feces. She then had a slight period of depression, and while depressed she inquired for her children and her husband for the first time in several weeks. Then she began to improve, and in about three months after her admission she became quiet, pleasant, and rational. She continued to gain steadily, and in a little less than four months from the date of admission she was discharged as recovered.

This case was remarkable for the violence of the mental manifestations, and the great physical unrest. It is considered a rather unfavourable symptom where the patient smears herself with feces, and yet in spite of that the case recovered. Though noisy and destructive and violent day and night for several weeks, she was nearly all the time good-natured. As we have said before, we have larger hopes for a patient who is cheerful in spirits than for one who is depressed and crying, or sullen, morose, or obstinate.

Hysterical Mania.—This form of mania is probably a prolonged exaggeration of some hysterical condition. Hysterical lunatics think they see visions of the Saviour and the Saints, and receive special messages in that way. Hysterical insane girls think they give birth to mice and frogs, and they also live on lime, and hair, and slate pencils. Sometimes they indulge in hysterical convulsions, in morbid waywardness, in ostentatious attempts at suicide, and in semivolitional retention of urine. Cases of hysterical insanity should be secluded from their friends, and trained and disciplined and cared for until they become stable in mind. (Clouston).

Disputed Forms of Mania

The disputed forms of mania, such as monomania, moral mania, and the manias of criminal tendencies, might all be classed under the general head of subacute mania. These cases are generally quiet and tractable when under discipline, and they cherish more or less the specific delusions which are characteristic of that form.

Under the influence of ideas of persecution or wrong, or impelled by a feeling that it is one's duty to rob, pillage or destroy, we have subacute maniacs who develop into kleptomaniacs or pyromaniacs. In such cases we find imbecility of the moral nature, together with a perversion of judgment, and an impairment of will power. In these cases the process of reasoning is at fault, the judgment is weak, the will erratic, and consequently the intellectual faculties bow before the fell influence of moral perversities. We must come, I believe, to consider insanity as a unit. There is a trinity of forces in man which tends to sane thought, moral speech, and rational action—namely, the physical, the intellectual, and the moral forces. If the physical force is vigorous, if the intellectual force is keen and clear, if the moral force is sensitive and true as the needle to the pole, then you will have sane thought, sane action, and sane conduct. These forces are united as closely, and as firmly interwoven as the Trinity of the Universe. When one is affected, the others, by contact or impression, are also affected. Break down the physical by disease, and you have perversions of both the intellectual and the moral forces. Hence we should dispense with the old-time dogma that a patient may be insane upon one point, and sane upon every other point. While this may appear to be the case, as a matter of fact if the man is insane upon one point, this taint of insanity affects generally his thoughts, and motives, and actions to a certain degree.

Pathological States

The pathology of mania is obscure, and as yet but little understood. The investigations of Edward Long Fox, M.D., F.R.C.P., in this direction have been carefully made, and we take pleasure in quoting briefly from his Pathological Anatomy of the nervous centers. He says: "Clinical observation, as well as pathological research, leads us to consider lesions of the vessels as at once the primary and the most important of all the cerebral changes in mania. It is this capillary distension, this hyperemia of the cortical substance of the brain, that is the chief lesion in acute mania. This hyperemia will generally affect the pia mater, and, I believe, especially the pia mater of the convexity."

Rindfleisch says that the cortical hyperemia will here cause a sort of stasis; this, again, leads to overdistension, then to atony of the vessels. This hyperemia of the pia mater and the cortex may be shown merely in a slight tinge of redness; more frequently, however, its previous presence is manifested by its results. These are extravasations, diffuse encephalitis, affecting especially one layer of the cortex, and pigmentation; and if the hyperemia has been long continued, or has frequently occurred, further changes are found to have taken place in the vessels themselves.

The extravasations may take the form of punctiform hemorrhages, but more usually the extravasation has not absolutely reached the brain matter, but exists in the form of dissecting aneurisms of the small veins. Besides these minute aneurisms we find various dilatations of the smallest vessels, causing alterations of shape of variable intensity. Dr. Bucknill thinks that in acute mania extravasations of blood are chiefly in the pia mater.

Greding states that "the choroid plexus was healthy in only 16 out of 216 cases of insanity, and that out of 100 maniacs 96 showed a choroid plexus that was either thickened or full of hydatids; by hydatids he doubtless meant serous cysts. The inflammatory condition met with in mania is usually confined to the middle layer of the cortex. The external layer is occasionally affected, this layer of the cortex coming off in patches when the pia mater is removed, and bearing the appearance of ragged ulcerations of the external portion of the brain." A similar condition exists when the brain of a general paretic is denuded of its pia mater covering, but from a different cause. In paresis there are inflammatory adhesions of the pia mater to the cortical substance, and when the former is peeled off it brings with it small particles of the cortex, leaving a brain surface which appears to have upon it *fine* ulcerations. In mania the second layer of cortical substance being somewhat softened, when the pia mater is removed there is sometimes the appearance of a rougher and more general breaking up of the convolutions of the brain than obtains in paresis. In paresis the particles that come away are like pin points; in mania the cortex, if it clings at all the pia mater, will be removed in patches.

Lecture VII

DEMENTIA

We shall today discuss that form of insanity known as Dementia. The term is derived from two Latin words, *de*, "from", and *mens*, "mind". The expression, therefore, means strictly "out of mind". It signifies, indeed, that the human being, thus bereft, is, to a considerable extent, in a state of the most deplorable mental poverty.

In discussing such a subject, we enter a field that is a vast desert waste. The paths across this field are strewn with the wrecks of early hopes, of joyous prospects, and of fruitless designs. The desert before us is a tiresome plain, unpeopled save by the ghostly images of uncertain recollection. Desolation is the ruling god of this desert, and destruction of mentality is his desperate and continued aim. And yet, in every desert there are some bright spots where, nourished by some hidden fountain, the perennial verdure springs. These gardens in the midst of the sand are called oases, and they signify that which is wonderful, and excellent, and unexpected. In the desert of dementia we have discovered some bright and hopeful spots. We have seen the light of recovery flash unexpectedly across the dark and gloomy pathway of some apparently hopeless victim. There are more oases in the distance awaiting attention, and Science, ever progressive, bears aloft her brilliant torch, lighting the path to future discoveries, and future amelioration of disease.

Esquirol states that dementia deprives men of the faculty of adequately perceiving objects, of seeing their relations to various things, of comparing them, or of preserving a complete recollection of them; whence results the impossibility of reasoning correctly. Demented persons are incapaable of reasoning because external objects make too feeble an impression upon them, because the organs of transmission have lost a part or all of their energy, or the brain itself has no longer sufficient strength to receive and retain the impression thus transmitted to it. Hence it necessarily results that the sensations are feeble, obscure and incomplete. Being unable to form a just and true idea of objects, these persons cannot compare them, or exercise abstraction or association of ideas. They are not capable of sufficiently strong attention; the organ of thought has not energy enough; it has been deprived of that vigor which is necessary for the integrity of its functions. Hence the most incongruous ideas succeed each other; they follow without order and without connection. It seems as if unreal expressions were whispered to them by unseen tongues, and these expressions are repeated by the patients in obedience to some involuntary or automatic impulse. Here we find examples of unconscious cerebration of a rare and interesting type, or rather a consciousness evolved from within and unrelated to association with external things, except through the medium of former impressions.

One great point of difference between dementia and idiocy and imbecility is that in both the latter the faculties are imperfect, while in the former they are simply enfeebled. Idiocy is a congenital absence of both cerebral and mental power. It is *amentia*, "without mind". Imbecility means a checked or arrested development. A child may have fair or moderate mental powers until the age of six, eight, ten or more years. Through disease or emotional disaster or injury, a shock is produced upon the nervous system, and this shock is sufficient to check all future mental growth. Hence an imbecile who is forty years of age will have the mind and capacity of a child of six or ten years of age. In fact, if a child becomes an imbecile at ten he will by and by only manifest the feeble powers of a child three or four years of age. That is, from the time the imbecility fairly begins there is a tendency toward degeneration. Still, there are some imbeciles who retain a special faculty for remembering names, or for adding up figures, or for playing upon some musical instruments. Now dementia, meaning "out of mind", is a condition of mental failure or infirmity, resulting after the mental powers have been developed or ripened to a fair extent. Dr. Winslow describes dementia as "a general enfeeblement of the intellect, and in some cases an apparent abolition of all mental powers". Mental power is always weakened in dementia, but comparatively seldom is that power utterly lost. We are speaking now of confirmed cases.

Dementia may be classified in a general way as primary and secondary. Primary dementia is a disease which comes on independently of any other form of insanity. Secondary dementia follows in the wake of some other form of insanity, chiefly melancholia or mania; and if this condition continues until the case is hopeless, it is then called terminal dementia.

Dementia may be either acute or chronic. That is, it may come on suddenly and with sharp manifestations, or it may gradually develop into a hopeless and long continued aberration.

Primary dementia may be sudden or gradual in its onset. Among the young and the poorly nourished, an attack of dementia is likely to be sudden, and then it is called acute primary dementia. Senile dementia (the dementia of old age) may be primary. That is, it may come on without any previous attack of any form of insanity, or it may come on so gradually that when actually observed and brought to the notice of the physician it is, to all intents and purposes, a chronic disease.

To primary and secondary dementias, with either acute or chronic tendencies, we may add, as special forms of this disease, masturbatic dementia, syphilitic dementia, epileptic dementia, organic dementia, alcoholic dementia, katatonic dementia, and senile dementia.

Causes and Symptoms of Acute Dementia

I now desire to call your attention to acute dementia, a form not common, but nevertheless interesting, because it affords under proper care strong hopes of recovery. It is to be distinguished from melancholia with stupor. The diagnostic differences were pointed out in my lecture on melancholia.

From the writings of J. Crichton Browne, as well as from our own observations, we learn that acute dementia attacks both sexes, but females in a larger proportion, though perhaps in a milder degree than males. It is essentially a disease of youth, being rarely seen in patients thirty years of age, and it seems, indeed, to be often dependent upon exhausting influences operating at a period of rapid growth. Children whose powers are overtaxed at a time when the process of development is going on, and when nutrition has not only to repair tissue waste, but is also obliged to contribute to the formation of new morphological elements, often fall into a state resembling idiocy, in which they are dull, sullen and depressed. And the children who are thus affected by acute dementia are not always those who have displayed extreme quickness of intellect, coupled with nervous instability, who have been clever and fragile, or who have inherited a predisposition to insanity. On the contrary, they are often those who have possessed only commonplace abilities, who have been robust dunces, and who have come of a perfectly healthy stock. For it is a peculiarity of acute dementia that it is less frequently connected with an hereditary taint than perhaps any other form of mental aberration. However diverse and multiplied the causes enumerated by some, we believe that neurotic tendencies have been assigned a prominent place among them; but that, perhaps, has arisen from force of habit rather than from accurate observation. Neurotic tendencies are the parents of such a multitude of evils that it seems one can scarcely be wrong in affiliating with them a malady having such a striking family resemblance to their acknowledged progeny. But minute inquiry will hardly warrant such a proceeding; for out of many recorded cases of acute dementia, the histories of which were satisfactorily traced, there were only about twenty-five per cent. in which an hereditary proclivity to mental or nervous diseases could be discovered. In most of the cases there was, so far as could be ascertained, an entire freedom from any such morbid impregnation.

It is not, of course, asserted that this disease may not have its roots in ancestral mold. What is alleged is that it far oftener grows out of superficial and individual conditions, and that they themselves are sufficient to account for its phenomena, without referring back to any hypothetical inheritance. Indeed, strange as it may sound, it has sometimes seemed that the absence of any neurotic inheritance was favorable to the development of acute dementia when its immediate causes come into play. These causes, such as debilitating occupations or insufficient nourishment, when operating upon neurotic subjects, have appeared to lead up to other disorders, to melancholia or mania, whereas, when acting upon more stolid beings, they have induced a blunting of the mental powers, or acute dementia.

It might be inferred, from what has just been said, that acute dementia is oftener due to physical than to moral causes, and that inference would be correct.

Moral impressions of a deleterious nature or intensity act more powerfully upon sensitive beings than upon those who are duller and steadier, and consequently they are not very influential over that class from which acute dements are drawn, unless physical conditions have previously produced prostration. Seldom do we hear of acute dementia being brought on by a fright, or a disappointment, or a joyous surprise, unless a state of extreme debility has existed when the emotional shock happened.

The one moral cause which is effectual in inducing this disorder is monotony of thought and feeling, or mental inanition. Man cannot live on bread alone. His dietary must be varied, and if it is not he becomes starved as effectually as if he were on short allowance. The human mind demands variety as the necessary and imperative spice of life, otherwise the mental forces fall into a condition of "innocuous desuetude". Under various conditions of life, where new impressions and ideas are not supplied, and where a tedious uninteresting routine is inevitable, does failure of mental power occur. This is especially the case when the deprivation of new impressions and the imposition of new restrictions are coincident with a period of mental evolution when the growing mind is greedy of nourishment suited to its wants.

Children who are sent at an early age into factories where they see brick walls and hear the same noises from machinery day after day and year after year, and where their work consists of muscular movements requiring close attention, often pass into a condition of acute dementia. Young prisoners in jail sometimes suffer in the direction of mental weakness from the wearisome monotony of their lives. Sailors stationed long at one place, where they experience simply the rolling of the ship and rumbling of the surf, become filled with a sense of tedium, and frequently have attacks of acute dementia. Factory life, prison life, and stationary sailor life are inimical to mental health, and tend to produce unnatural weakness of the faculties. But the failure of brain force must not be charged to one cause alone. The majority of such cases arise, not only from monotonous existence, but also from being poorly fed and indifferently housed. A lowered vitality caused by poor food and hard work prepares the victim most surely for the inception and growth of this grave malady.

Acute diseases, such as typhoid and other fevers, have sometimes acute dementia among their sequelæ. It is also brought on occasionally by protracted diarrhea, by bleeding piles, by leucorrhea, by menorrhagia, or by any severely exhausting and depleting disease. It may even derive its origin from malaria or atmospheric miasma. It follows also in the wake of alcoholism, gluttony, and masturbation, even as sharks follow ships that have corpses on board.

But however induced, acute dementia makes its actual invasion in one of two ways:

(1) It either steals over the patient by gradual and at first almost imperceptible encroachments for a few days; or (2) it is ostentatiously ushered in by an attack of excitement. In the first case some slips of memory, some relaxations of attention, some expression of wandering thoughts, some moments of blank bewilderment, are its earliest harbingers; while in the second case an outbreak of fury, wild bursts of laughter, swift meaningless movements of the arms

DEMENTIA

and head, and the giving forth of broken disconnected sentences are the symptoms which announce its presence.

When once established in any way this disease manifests itself by a greater or less suspension of the psychical activities. Impressions are slowly transmitted to the mind, and are imperfectly assimilated, so that only a dim knowledge is obtained of external things or events by the victim of dementia. Comparison is suspended, imagination has abandoned its creative work, desire which in health surges so tumultuously in the human breast now scarcely moves within. Affections and passions are dormant, and the will is destitute of strength. This inward mental inability is outwardly expressed in modifications of physiognomy, in gait, and in conduct. The countenance wears a perplexed and vacant expression; the attitude betokens lethargy or irresolution; the voice loses its accustomed tone, and the limbs perform their duties with uncertain effort. The patient is sullen and self-absorbed. If spoken to, he gives no heed to what is said. His memory becomes impaired; his command of language is reduced to the minimum; he performs his work, if at all, in a slovenly and careless way. Most frequently all labors are given up, and all exercises are renounced. At this stage some curious exhibitions of the imitative faculty and automatic muscular activity are sometimes seen. A girl acutely demented was asked repeatedly and forcibly: "What is your name?" Being awakened and stirred into activity, she at last cried out "Elizebeth", and from the time for a whole month foliowing, when spoken to, she screamed "Elizabeth". In the same way, if patients of this class are made to walk or run, they will continue to exercise automatically until they are stopped. A patient will sometimes feed herself in this way: A plate filled with chopped up food is put in the proper position, a spoon is put into the patient's hand, and then the patient is made to dip the spoon into the food and convey it to her mouth. After doing this a few times, she will go on automatically and empty the plate. (Browne).

When acute dementia is of a severe type, the mental state becomes one of profound stupidity. Comparison is abolished, memory is a blank, language is lost, the sentiments are lifeless, the will is palsied, and even the normal wants are not attended to. Organic existence alone remains. The sufferer is indifferent to all that is taking place around him. Pricking or pinching the skin does not cause signs of pain, nor does tickling produce responsive movements. The patient will sit or stand for hours in one position, lacking spontaneity of purpose to change it. Now and then a species of catalepsy is observed in these cases. The limbs remain for a time in any position in which they may be placed; the body in any attitude in which it may be thrown. If the arms are raised above the head they will be held there perhaps for an hour. Such an effort would cause intense suffering to a healthy person, and yet in these demented cases there is no great rigidity of the muscles. The limbs are flaccid, and are readily flexed and extended, and it is remarkable that after being long held in positions in which great resistance to gravitation must be exerted, they are still free from stiffness.

Of the bodily symptoms of acute dementia, those connected with the circulatory system are most prominent. They consist of feeble action of the heart, small and almost imperceptible pulse at the wrist, and passive congestion of the extremities. The hands and feet are cold, and have a bluish-red color, which disappears under pressure, leaving a patch of pale skin; but the color speedily returns when the pressure is removed. This coldness and blueness is very striking, and is often accompanied by considerable swelling.

The hands and feet are sometimes affected by diffuse chilblains which form and persist even during summer, and when the extremities are kept warm, and wrapped in cotton wool. There is often edema of the joints. The face has a puffed and livid appearance. When excitement comes on in the mind of the dement, there is generally active flushing of the face and heat of the head. The pupils in acute dementia are more or less dilated, and somewhat inactive. The respiration is quite shallow; sometimes the patient can scarcely be seen to breathe. In advanced stages of the disease, there is liability to edema of the lungs. The temperature in the axilla or rectum is generally about normal, but in the chilled hands it has been known to fall as much as ten or fifteen degrees, Fahrenheit, below the normal standard. The tongue is tolerably clean; sometimes swollen and pale in color, and bears the imprints of the teeth at the edges. (Browne and others). There is almost always a copious flow of saliva, and sometimes the amount secreted and poured out is very great. As much as a pint of saliva has been collected in five hours from one case—a very fair record of sap exudation from a human maple tree! The appetite is generally good, if pains are taken to feed the patient properly. Now and then the food is rejected, but with as little sign of nausea or emotion as a child manifests when it throws off its surplus of milk. The bowels are frequently constipated, but occasionally an exhausting diarrhea supervenes. In females who are attacked with acute dementia there is generally amenorrhea, and sometimes leucorrhea; but the process of excretion from the membranes, except the mouth, seems to be checked. The female patient is apt to become excited at the time when the menstrual flux should occur.

Upon recovering from acute dementia, the patient finds a great hiatus or vacancy in his memory. He has passed through the "valley of the shadow of death", and the shades have rested like a black mantle upon his mind. His soul has been laved in the sullen waters of Lethe, and perfect oblivion of his sufferings is the fortunate result. In melancholia with stupor, you will recollect, the melancholiac is cognizant of every event, and remembers with clearness the details of his perilous voyage through the tideless, and sunless, and moonless slough of despond.

While we shall in a subsequent lecture enlarge upon the treatment of these cases, we may tell you here that the prone position in bed, to favor easy circulation, and an abundant liquid diet, warm clothing, and appropriate medication, are essential to successful treatment.

Chronic Dementia.—We come now to consider the phases of chronic dementia.

> "Last scene of all,
> That ends this strange eventful history,
> Is second childishness and mere oblivion,
> Sans teeth, sans eyes, sans taste, sans everything."

The "sans everything" to which Shakespeare alludes is the sad and hopeless obscuration by time or disease of the once bright, vigorous, scintillating mental powers of exuberant and lusty youth.

Ben Jonson was once called upon to admire a beautiful palace, but he growled at his companion and urged him to hurry on, saying: "It is the sight of such things as these that makes death horrible." A contemplation of the ravages of dementia excites a horror of existence, for it reveals a life full of grand possibilities shorn at the last of every vestige of mental cheer; and it proves with crucial force that living with such deprivations in prospect is a most solemn and trying thing. It is a solemn thing to die, but, as

Mrs. Partington says, "it is a good deal solemner to live". But when we are brought face to face with the unfortunate physical wrecks of humanity, we are compelled by duty not to shrink, but to examine carefully the sources of the wreck, and to patch it up, and make it more comfortable and habitable for its spiritual occupant, if possible.

After the disappearance of a severe attack of acute mania, the effects of the shock are sometimes visible in a certain condition of mental weakness without actual intellectual disorder. The force of character seems to have been snapped, and the finer moral and esthetic feelings, which are the bloom of culture, are abolished. The physiognomy has lost its highest expression, and the individual presents the appearance of a certain childishness. This is one end of the scale of degeneration, but at the other the mental powers are almost obliterated, the acquisitions of the past being completely blotted out. There is no interest in the present, and the patient leads a merely vegetative life. Between these two extremes of slow weakness on the one hand, and absolute mental failure on the other, we note every shade of transition from strength to helplessness.

The countenance of the chronic dement no longer expresses any fixed passion. There is a want of harmony, or, as it were, a dislocation of the features, and the most that is manifested is the shivered expression of a passion, or the shattered wreck of a smile. There is a corresponding imbecility on the motor side. Some can continue their former occupation, or can do a little simple manual work; but there is no sharp energy impelling to action. Not infrequently the industrious breadwinner of a large family concludes, in a condition of dementia, his busy industry on earth, by gathering bits of stone, or pieces of glass, or wood, or any small, light, movable objects that come in his way. Strange propensities of all kinds are exhibited, as, for example, to sit on the floor doubled up like a jack knife, to stand or crouch in a particular corner, to walk backward and forward for a certain distance on a particular strip of ground, to fantastically ornament the person with feathers or flowers, or to repeat some particular phrase. A patient will get hold of a delusion and repeat it automatically for days, and weeks, and years. Hallucinations and illusions of the extremest kind are frequent, and tend to sustain the delusion. One woman nurses as her child a lump of wood decked in rags; another person, whose singular movements seem unaccountable, is busy spinning threads out of sunbeams, while a third continues the most violent movements of his arm in order to prevent the motion of the universe, or of his own blood from coming to a stand. The mood may be of surly depression or of more or less exaltation.

The bodily health is usually good, the patient frequently getting stout as the active symptoms of mania or melancholia subside into the calm of dementia. Some patients suffering with chronic dementia may be made to work, but they require most careful guidance.

The end of chronic dementia is usually death. Occasionally a recovery takes place during the onset of some acute disease. One case of four years' standing and apparently hopelessly demented, recovered his mental powers during a severe attack of tonsillitis. During this attack his temperature ran up to 105°F, and he became delirious and talked in a rambling and muttering manner. The inflammatory conditions were remarkably intense. When they subsided, the mind was clear, and the patient talked quietly and rationally. He continued to improve for several months, and finally recovered and returned to his home, and resumed his work as a blacksmith.

This man's memory of events which occurred during his dementia was completely obliterated. He experienced four years of mental obfuscation. After recovery, his memory of facts and events, which had been presented to his mind before his illness, was as clear and strong as ever.

We have dwelt at some length upon acute and chronic dementia. We will now consider, briefly, some of the special forms of dementia due to particular or specific causes.

Masturbatic Dementia.—This form of insanity is a result of that perversive and brain-impairing vice familiarly known as "self-abuse". Sometimes a person addicted to this unfortunate habit will suffer with remorse to the extent of developing mild or acute melancholia. And again, the victim of masturbation may pass into a condition resembling subacute mania, where the patient is sullen, irritable, suspicious, and often thinks himself the victim of some conspiracy or plot to injure him. But all cases of masturbatic insanity eventually terminate in dementia, unless cured or relieved of this deplorable habit.

In patients suffering with masturbatic dementia, we find, as a rule, but very moderate intellectual powers, and especially are the forces of the will weak and erratic in their operations. The animal propensities are strong and unrestrained. These persons are frequently of a religious cast of mind. Indeed, one of our patients thus afflicted was in the habit of saying his prayers, and of masturbating at the same time. It may seem almost sacrilegious to refer to such a fact, but it is proper that you, as physicians, should be put upon your guard, and when you suspect a given case of masturbating, you should not be diverted from your investigations by the assurances of the parents that the boy "is very good, and says his prayers regularly".

The treatment of masturbatic insanity must be moral,

medical, dietetic, and hygienic. The proper course to pursue is to carefully examine the sexual organs, for the purpose of discovering abnormalities, and if such exist an operation should be performed. The boy should be circumcised, while, if necessary, the hood should be removed from the clitoris of the girl. Then by keeping the parts clean, the source of irritation may be dispensed with, and the disposition to masturbate may be cured.

These patients should be taught the folly of their actions, and at the same time they should be made to feel that such an unwise use of God-given powers does not constitute the unpardonable sin, nor preclude the possibility of recovery and usefulness. They should be encouraged by their family physician to leave off bad habits, and likewise to abstain from too much remorse.

Those addicted to unfortunate personal habits are generally seclusive, and inclined to hide away from everybody, especially from those of the opposite sex. The lives and the habits of such patients should be changed. They should be lifted from their settled grooves of thought and action. They should be taken from their books, their prayers, and their solitude, and placed among genial and active people of both sexes. These patients often profess a great love for books. They retire to their rooms or to some secluded forest shade ostensibly for study, but in reality to indulge in lecherous imaginings, lewd thoughts, salacious efforts, and peccant practices. They should not be allowed to dream or dawdle themselves into dementia, but they should be stirred in other directions, and elevated to better and nobler things. Their energies should be restrained, and stored up for future drafts established by the wise and glorious economy of nature. Farming, herding cattle on horseback, engaging in railroad enterprises, mining, or any work that is hard and reasonably exhausting to the physical forces, are the proper channels of toil for such cases. Outdoor air, both in sunshine and in storm, is a necessity; and plenty of plain food, and a hard bed to sleep on at night, and constant association with those who are clear-headed and watchful, are likewise demanded.

Syphilitic Dementia.—This form of dementia sometimes supervenes among those who have led fast and disreputable lives. These cases are generally hopeless, although death and other unfavorable symptoms may be postoned or mitigated by appropriate medication. Syphilitic dements usually have gummy deposits or tumors in the brain. These may produce, besides loss of memory or loss of sight, paralysis of one or both sides of the body, and finally a series of convulsions in which the patient dies. It is said that almost every case of epileptiform seizure occurring after the age of forty is due to a neurosis dependent upon syphilis. Traumatic injury may, of course, produce some cases of epilepsy after middle life.

Epileptic Dementia.—Epileptic dementia frequently follows a long continued series of epileptic fits. Victims of epilepsy are quite apt to be depressed or melancholy at times or again maniacal in their speech and action. But at last they nearly all become more or less demented. Such cases require close care, good nursing, light diet, and such sympathy as their helpless and deplorable state demands.

Organic Dementia.—Organic dementia is an enfeeblement of the mental powers, complicated with or supervening upon a paralysis of one or both sides of the body. It is usually a disease of middle or advanced life. It follows frequently an attack of apoplexy, or it may occur after long continued gluttony or drunkenness. It may arise from syphilitic or other tumors of the brain. It may owe its origin to excessive sexual indulgence, or to excessive care, anxiety or overwork. Even an uncontrolled fit of anger might induce it. Organic dementia is the result of a marked and positive brain lesion. Therefore but little hope of a permanent recovery may be indulged in. However, as the lesion is commonly local, it may, with good care, be partially relieved. Nature is always on hand after every local injury to the system with a powerful "work gang", and the task of repair and clearing up the debris is sometimes happily and unexpectedly accomplished. Even if the channels of thought and action are clogged, new channels may be opened. Collateral circulation may take up and perform successfully the work of nourishment, even where a main artery has been plugged by an obstructing embolus. Hence we should be unremitting in our efforts to relieve cases of organic dementia, for some cases may be materially helped, although the vast majority can never recover.

Alcoholic Dementia.—This form of dementia is produced by the protracted use of alcoholic stimulant. In this form the failure of mental power is not so marked as in some other forms; but the deplorable feature in these cases is that the disease is self-induced, is largely avoidable, and, worst of all, it strikes down some of the strongest and best men the world has ever known.

Remedies for the relief of alcoholic dementia are of little avail so long as the exciting cause continues; yet a too sudden withdrawal of long continued accustomed stimuli might result, in some instances, in a still deeper dementia. Therefore, the physician in treating such patients needs profoundest wisdom and ripest judgment if he would do what is really best for his case. Probably the wiest thing you can do for the welfare of the community is to warn the young against excesses of all kinds. The last and bitterest result of overindulgence in strong drinks, or in any other excess, is an engulfment in the yawning pitfall of dementia.

Katatonic Dementia.—Patients affected with this form of dementia repeat constantly and deliberately the same sentence or phrase. For instance, No. 1659 says: "I think my name is E. E. W. My own dear mother, who was kind and faithful to me for many years, that was my own precious mother from my birth for many years, that took faithful care of me for many years, called me sometimes Libbie, and I think my name is Elizabeth. My own dear father, who was kind and faithful to me for many years, sometimes called me Libbie. I think I do not promise to stay in this room. I don't think it necessary for me to marry any man. A woman told me I must not marry any man".

Senile Dementia.—Senile dementia is the result of both old age and of acquired cerebral disease. It should be carefully distinguished from simple old age or dotage. In the latter case the mind is weakened, but the patient is clearly conscious of his own weakness. He forgets a name or a date, and gropes about in his memory to find it. The dement is not conscious of loss of memory, but applies wrong names to persons, and serenely thinks he is right. Senile dementia is something more than the mere loss of mental power which results from the natural decay of the faculties. It is complicated also with those pathological changes which are essential to the production of insanity. It does not consist alone in the enfeeblement of the faculties, because if it did we would find that every old man is a victim of senile dementia. There are several stages or degrees of it. In the first occurs a loss of memory, particularly of recent events, without any serious impairment of the reasoning faculties. Early impressions and ideas long retained now come up fresh from their resting place. From forgetfulness of recent events, accompanied by recollections of early ones, occur many of those gaps in ideas and incoherence that, in part, constitute dementia. This defect, or loss of memory, generally marks the commencement of dementia from this cause, but not invariably. Sometimes it begins with nervous erethism, accompanied by the excitement of some faculty, function, or active power, which may act with great energy. Some become irritated by the slightest circumstance; others experience venereal desires long since extinguished; while others still, of regular, temperate and sober habits, all at once manifest an appetite for highly seasoned dishes and intoxicating drinks. These symptoms are soon succeeded by those of absolute dementia.

The second degree is characterized by a loss of the reasoning power. Either the reflective faculties are so completely impaired that they are unable to exercise their functions, or the other faculties are so completely prolapsed that normal functions are no longer exercised. The emotional faculties are so much enfeebled that the will does not possess sufficient strength and energy to carry out any process of reasoning. The premises are scarcely laid down before they are forgotten. Hence the inability to draw conclusions from them. The transaction of any business which requires a sustained attention becomes impossible. Any slight or irrelevant idea in disturbing the attention draws the mind away from what it was considering, and thus destroys all attempts at continuous effort. Some individuals in this stage recognize their friends, but seldom manifest any signs of emotion on seeing them.

The next stage, or third degree, is termed "incomprehension", and is attended by an inability to comprehend the meaning of any principle or proposition, however simple, that is proposed. Attention, memory, reason, all but the mere instincts, are entirely lost. Here is sometimes found a great degree of physical activity, such as jumping, running, or walking. Some talk unmeaning jargon; others mutter half sentences or broken expressions; while others are found sitting in silence, scarcely pronouncing a syllable for weeks, months, or even years.

The fourth and last degree consists in a loss of instinctive action. The mode of existence is merely organic. There is neither desire nor aversion, hardly a consciousness of life.

One more point concerning dementia. You may be called upon in the courts to give evidence as to the testamentary capacity of a person suffering with dementia. To do this justly, you must be able to distinguish between dotage (old age) and dementia. In both cases there is weakness of the mental powers, but the victim of old age is, as I have already said, cognizant of that fact. The senile dement does not realize his condition, and more than this, if any mental power is left he cherishes delusions or false beliefs on account of the imperfect or erroneous impressions received by his disordered senses. A clear statement of facts as you discover them by a cautious examination, and by a careful diagnosis between the mental weakness of age and the mental obliquity of brain disease, may enable you to conserve the ends of justice.

Pathological States

The blood vessels of the bodies of acute dements, and especially the capillaries and veins, are dilated, and their walls relaxed. The circulation throughout is languid and sluggish. The general condition of the mind is that of relaxation and obfuscation.

The pathological state of the brain of chronic dements may be best described by the term "cerebral chilblains"

There is atony and dilatation of the veins of the pia mater; the arachnoid becomes thickened and opaque; while the dura mater is but little changed. The general condition is too sluggish to produce any marked pathological impression upon the dura mater, which is a tough membrane. The frontal and parietal lobes are water-logged upon the surface, and wasted within. The gray matter is paler than usual, and the brain substance is tumid, spongy, and edematous. The stasis or clogging of the circulatory apparatus of the brain readily accounts for the marked mental failure.

The pathological conditions induced by the excessive use of alcohol are thickening of the membranes, slow serous effusions, atrophy of the cerebral substance, with sclerosis or hardening of the tissue.

Lecture VIII

GENERAL PARESIS

We invite your attention today to the last general form or division of insanity—namely, General Paresis. This formidable and fatal disease is a cosmopolitan type of all modern insanity, and represents to the fullest degree the effects of toil, worry, and intemperance in every shade and form. It is a deep-seated, far-reaching, intractable scourge which fastens its fangs upon the matured brains of its victim, and it rarely, if ever, yields up its hold.

Early in the nineteenth century Esquirol made note of the fact that a person suffering with insanity complicated with paralysis was not likely to recover. In 1822, Bayle made some successful observations of the disease, and outlined its description. In 1826, Calmeil, a French physician, first intelligently and carefully described the disease known as general paresis. Not until 1843 did Dr. Luther B. Bell, of the McLean Asylum, near Boston, discover it in this country. He reported several cases of the disease, all of which died. In 1847, Dr. Pliny Earle, at that time of the Bloomingdale Asylum, gave to the profession a few more cases of the disease; and about the same time Dr. Brigham, of the State Hospital at Utica, detected and described the so-called new malady.

Much has been written upon this same subject since its first discovery. Probably the fullest and most notable work upon General Paralysis of the Insane is by William Julius Mickle, M.D., M.R.C.P., London.

But while modern doctors have studied the disease very fully, and while they have written much upon this subject, no one has more concisely described the disorder and its inevitable termination than Shakespeare. Nearly three centuries ago, this great polychrest of thinkers and observers wrote, concerning the then undiscovered paretic:

> "Things small as nothing, for request's sake only,
> He makes important: possess'd he is with greatness;
> And speaks not to himself, but with a pride
> That quarrels at self-breath: imagined worth
> Holds in his blood such swoll'n and hot discourse,
> That, 'twixt his mental and his active parts,
> Kingdom'd Achilles in commotion rages,
> And batters 'gainst itself. What should I say?
> He is so plaguy proud, that the death-tokens of it
> Cry—*No recovery*."
>
> *Troilus and Cressida*, Act, II, Sc. 3

The synonyms of general paresis are: General paralysis, general progressive paralysis, general paralysis of the insane, *mania de gandeur*, and dementia paralytica or paralytic dementia. The latter term might more appropriately be applied either to the last stage of this general disease, or to a condition of both mental and physical loss following apoplexy, embolism, or thrombosis.

Just here we wish to define the difference which we conceive to exist between paresis and paralysis. The latter term implies a loss of the powers of motion, either complete or partial. Accompanying this loss, there is frequently an impairment of sensation as well. Paralysis is from the Greek, παρλνω, "I loosen". Paresis is from the Greek, παριημι, "I relax", and means a relaxation of the nerves of motion. In its effects upon these nerves it differs in degree from paralysis. Through the influence of paresis the nerves become less "taut" than natural, and the result is a certain tremulousness of the muscles controlling the organs of speech, and a general inaccuracy in the movements of the

GENERAL PARESIS

arms and legs. The nerves respond to every impulse for action, but in a lax and hesitating manner, just as the strings of a violin give forth imperfect sounds when they are but partially tightened. In paralysis there is no response to impulse of the will in the affected parts. Some one or all of the strings in the human violin are completely unstrung or broken.

STAGES

General paresis may be divided into four stages, namely:

1. The incipient or irritable stage; the stage of worrry, anxiety, sleeplessness, and melancholy.

2. The well-defined stage of the disease; the stage of maniacal excitement, and of active delusions of wealth, of power, and of grandeur, alternating in some cases with attacks of temporary depression.

3. The stage of subsidence, when the patient passes into a condition of subacute or chronic mania, with a general but slow tendency toward decadence.

4. The stage of terminal dementia, of physical as well as mental failure, and of death.

The first stage is usually marked by a long continued and suspicious prodrome. The man who has been active and hopeful in appearance, yet withal concealing an undercurrent of worry and anxiety, becomes at last unable, through the effects of subtle disease, to carry on concealment any longer. The disease has robbed him of his natural carefulness.

The prospective victim of paresis worries more than is his usual custom. Gradually his sleep is shortened, and disturbed by anxious dreams. The tendency to sleeplessness and anxiety may be accompanied by a sense of heaviness and fullness in the brain, and this frequently extends to the degree of positive pain, although some paretics assert that they never had a headache. Still, the brain changes which are observed after death would indicate that the pains of slow, subacute inflammation have been experienced.

From sleeplessness, melancholy, anxiety, and worriment, the patient passes through the heaviness of mental abstraction, until he suddenly loses self-control, and indulges in outbursts of anger. The depressed and irritable stage is passed usually in a few weeks or months, although this condition may last two or three years before the upheaval of maniacal excitement. In some cases the physical symptoms of paresis are present, and the patient passes from a condition of melancholy to a state of dementia without being called upon to endure the excitement occasioned by the cherishing of delusions of wealth and grandeur.

Even in the melancholic stage it will be observed that the paretic is more earnestly engaged in projecting enterprises than heretofore. In doing so he loses his ordinary prudence in the affairs of life. He also forgets the principle of right and wrong, and sometimes becomes a thief, because he thinks everything he can lay hands on is his own property. The blunting of the perceptions of justice, and truth, and right, and honor is one of the first evidences of approaching paresis.

Having passed through the stage of worry, anxiety, depression, and loss of the moral sense, the patient finally develops full-grown delusions of wealth, and power, and grandeur. At this stage the natural affections of the man seem to fail. The normal common sense having departed, the paretic indulges in wild and extravagant purchases, or in unwarrantable business schemes. He begins to feel "first-rate", and yet he is evidently failing; and also he becomes tremulous in body, and unsteady in mental action

GENERAL PARESIS

The physician who is called to see an active paretic in the early maniacal stage will probably discover some of the following indications:

1. The pupils are either unequally dilated (one being larger than usual, while the other may be contracted), or the pupils may be equally dilated, or equally contracted. But in either case they are irresponsive to light, that is, the motor muscles of the pupil do not respond quickly and naturally to the stimulus of light. Irresponsiveness to light, on the part of the pupils, is characteristic of nearly every case of general paresis.

2. The patient is unable to control the motions of the eye. There is a certain restlessness and unsteadiness in moving the eye which, to a careful observer, is often discernible. Of course, people suffering with chorea, or paralysis agitans, or some other nerve disorder, may suffer with eye twitchings; but the history of their cases will eliminate them from a consideration of paresis.

3. A dropping of one corner of the mouth is sometimes seen, owing to a partial paralysis of the facial nerve.

4. There is a marked tremulousness of the lips and tongue. This tremulousness of the paretic should be diagnosed from that of acute drunkenness, or mental excitement.

5. A slight hesitancy of speech is apparent, as well as a deliberate attempt to overcome this inability to articulate clearly.

6. There is a tendency to stammering, especially when using words in which the letters k, l, m, r, and e occur.

7. There is a slight unsteadiness of gait, that is, the patient has a shambling uncertain step as if the knees were tired, and the owner could not determine which way to bend them.

8. There is a smoothing out or a partial obliteration of the natural lines of intelligence in the face.

9. The skin presents a sallow and wax-like appearance, and sometimes feels as if it were greasy. Greasiness and flabbiness are characteristic of the skin conditions of the paretic.

10. A slight exaltation of temperature. The temperature of a paretic often runs from one-half to two degrees above the normal, and during a convulsive seizure, to which he becomes liable, the temperature may go much higher.

These are some of the physical signs of paresis in the active stage. Mentally, there is an intense disturbance of the imagination. Visions of boundless wealth are conjured up in the overwrought mind of the patient. A sense of power, the most magnificent, pervades his every thought. He himself is the greatest and strongest man and financier in the world. (Women paretics have delusions about gold and diamonds, rich clothing, numerous children, fine houses, and grand carriages. Women paretics do not often attempt to make money. They simply endeavor to spend what has already been made). The expansive delusions are contrary to the natural belief of the patient. Generally the victims of paresis are plain, hard-working, common sense individuals, although they may be mercurial and ardent in temperament, and ambitious to get on in the world.

Under the influence of his mighty projects, the paretic loses the power of considering the common affairs of life. He forgets familiar names. He fails to remember recent dates of appointments. He also loses the power of calculating. His delusions multiply and reduplicate fortunes in geometrical order, while the forces of the mind, as applied to common things, diminish in arithmetical ratio. Some paretics make little account of immense fortunes, but they fancy themselves the possessors of numberless wives, or they see themselves able to drink innumerable flagons of wine. But whether the current of thought is toward strong drink, or seductive sirens, or Croesus-like wealth, it is a current that is forever widening and deepening until its unfortunate burden is cast into eternity.

Sometimes, at irregular intervals, between his fitful visions of unearthly grandeur, the paretic patient sinks into the gloomy abyss of melancholy. There are days when he weeps easily, and sends up a wail of anxiety and hopelessness which contrasts with his customary lofty and exuberant spirits as the mournful strains of the Dead March in Saul contrast with the sublimer sweeps and surges of the Hallelujah Chorus.

As the active paretic indulges in delusions of strength and wealth, so he is likely to use the ordinary courses of business transactions with which to develop not only his special projects, but also to reveal his mental condition. The paretic patient will often write scores of letters or telegrams in a single day. He is always in an intolerable hurry to accomplish his work; therefore he seeks to use the telegraph and the fast mail for the purpose of accomplishing his ends. It is an interesting fact that the more excitable an insane person becomes, the larger and more irregular are the letters which he makes. In addition to making the letters large, the patient in writing often omits words, or letters from words. This may occur from inattention, and from the hurry to get through the task. Occasionally the patient will adorn his rhetoric by gaudy illustrations with colored pencils. When the excitement subsides, and the patient becomes quiet and calm, he will often resume, to a certain extent, his natural style of writing; that is, the letters will be formed upon a more moderate plan, but the words or parts of words may still be omitted. The paretic uses so much force and ink in the construction of his letters, and is so anxious to finish them, that they are often marred and blotted.

From the state of active delusion and active exertion, the patient passes slowly and surely into what may be termed the chronic state of paresis, which is marked by an exaggeration of all physical weaknesses, and a subsidence of the delusions, with occasional flashes of excitement or attacks of depression. The unsteadiness of gait becomes more pronounced; the tremulousness of lips and tongue is strikingly apparent; the patient is careless of dress and person, and in every way we note a decadence of physical and mental powers. Sometimes the appetite in this stage is enormous, and the patient takes on loads of fat. This soon passes away, and leaves the patient thinner than ever. The march of the disease may be interrupted by an episode of epileptiform convulsions, at which time partial paralysis may occur. These attacks are often brief, the paralysis lasting only a few hours or days.

After an attack of these convulsions, the patient loses ground rapidly. The mind fails, and dementia supervenes. The appetite is capricious, the physical strength wanes, the body emaciates, and the nerves atrophy. The skin, which has been flabby, sticky, and clammy, is now apt to break out in eruptions known as pemphigus foliaceus. At first these large watery blebs are noticed on the extremities; afterward there is superficial ulceration of the derma, followed by scabbing and attempts at healing. These sores heal slowly, if at all. It is one of the most remarkable features of this strange disease that the patient may continue to live long after all the forces of life appear to be exhausted, and when little remains but the skeleton, overlaid by a parchment-like and very ragged skin. Of course we are now describing an extreme case, though many of this kind have come under our observation and care during the past twenty-five years. Relief from life comes at last through utter exhaustion. Sometimes for several hours previous to dissolution, the patient becomes unconscious and thus passes away. With others, consciousness remains until very near the end, and with the last articulate breath of conscious life the dying man, corrugating his countenance into a ghastly smile, will reply to your inquiries as to how he feels today with the stock expression, "fuss rate".

The pulse of paretics is soft and weak. This is due to the relaxation of the muscular coats of the arteries, and probably relaxation of the heart itself. Every portion of the paretic's body is, to a greater or less extent, relaxed and unable to perform normal duty. The stomach and bowels partake of the general relaxation, and the food is often passed undigested. Lack of assimilation of food accounts for the gradually increasing weakness and exhaustion which this disease produces.

There is sometimes danger to paretic patients in the act of eating, for they cram their mouths so full of food at times as to almost suffocate. The muscles of deglutition, also, being relaxed and eccentric or uncertain in action, will sometimes suddenly fail, and a patient will choke to death by the impaction of food in the larynx. When a patient is inclined to eat voraciously and rapidly, he should be fed carefully by an attendant, and his food should be of a liquid or semi-liquid nature.

The paretic patient will sometimes grind his teeth by the hour or by the day, and this is thought to be a diagnostic symptom by some. But cases of acute delirious mania will often grind their teeth, and so will some cases of chronic dementia.

That you may see how naturally the actual facts in given cases coincide with the pen picture which we have presented, we will now give a few condensed extracts from the records of the hospital under my charge. The histories which we shall reveal will bring you face to face with grim and sad realities.

P. B., æt. 50, married. Symptoms of mental derangement had been well marked for nine months previous to admission. For many years Mr. B. had been engaged in business requiring a severe mental strain. He was a man of excellent and methodical habits, and strictly temperate, save in matters of over-work and worry. Previously to the attack of paresis his health had been good. In temperament, he was of the nervous order. In disposition, he was hasty and impulsive, although kind, and from principle, carefully self-controlled. Three years before admission to the hospital, however, it was noticed that he became unusually overbearing in his manner, and for one year prior to admission was subject to nocturnal excitement. During the previous summer he was attacked with melancholy, which was followed by a maniacal outburst.

When admitted, Mr. B. was in good bodily health, although he was not sleeping well. The only thing he complained of was a necessity for passing his water somewhat too frequently. He was very restless, and spent his time walking up and down the hall, talking to himself, and taking no notice of any one. He claimed that his wife had been unfaithful to him; and he also entertained the delusion that the attic of the hospital building was stored with chests of gold belonging to him. He worried and talked so much about this, that he was finally taken to the attic and allowed to examine it, and was greatly disappointed at not finding any trace of the treasure. Ordinarily he complained of no pain, and considered himself perfectly well. For sometime this patient continued his active exercise during the day, and slept but little at night. After a time, when appearing quite well, he admitted that his only brain trouble was "forgetfulness". Most of the time, however, he cherished and manifested delusions concerning persons and events. At one time he indulged in great railroad schemes, and was going to build an elevated twelve-track road between all the large cities in this country. This road was to be placed upon trestle work two hundred feet in height. Again, he had the delusion, which he disclosed every day for several weeks, that there were nine hundred, or more, headless bodies in the basement of the building in which he was located. Again, he expressed very seriously a wish to exchange heads with some one. And again, he projected the idea of starting an immense printing office which would contain five hundred mammoth Hoe presses with which he would do all the printing in New York City. While engaged in these mighty projects, with the idea constantly in mind that he could accomplish each one of these chimercial enterprises, his memory was rapidly failing. He became so weak in this respect that he could not remember even the names of his constant attendants. He would ask the same questions over and over many times in the course of a few minutes. At length he came to have hallucinations of hearing, and would frequently talk to imaginary persons. Physically, he varied; at times eating ravenously, and taking on much flabby flesh; at other times failing in appetite, and correspondingly losing in weight. It was noticed that he went often to urinate, and that he drank large quantities of water. He was watched on account of these peculiarities, and it was observed that during ten hours he urinated eleven times, and drank copious draughts from the water tank seventeen times, beside drinking much at meals. It was estimated that he sometimes drank between three and four gallons of water in a single day. At such times he would consume with his food large quantities of salt, pepper, and vinegar. His friends, failing to secure from us any favourable prognosis, determined to try a change of treatment. He was taken to a water cure for a few days, and then transferred to the care of a distinuished old school physician in Connecticut who declared, so we were told by the friends, "that the case was not by any means incurable". He continued, however, to run down, and died about a year and a half later.

In this case you will observe that the cause was neither intemperance nor sexual excess, but simply mental strain from business cares and worry. Also there may possibly have been some hereditary taint, which we believe to be unusual in such cases. The father and mother, brothers and sisters, were always mentally sound, but a maternal aunt was reported as insane. The delusions in this case were marked, and sleeplessness was a symptom, though many paretics sleep well. The patient drank large quantities of water without having any marked fever, a symptom which we have observed in quite a number of cases. In no other non-febrile disease is there likely to be such ravenous thirst as in paresis.

J. A., æt. 41, married, but had no children. The disease had been gradually making its appearance for about six months. The assigned cause was intemperance or fast living. Our prognosis was unfavourable from the outset. The friends gave as the history of the case that the patient had been "irritable and strange-acting" for about six months; that he had been a hard drinker for a long time, and very ardent in the performance of marital duties. During the two weeks previous to admission he had been reckless, violent and unmanageable. This excitement continued, and in fact increased after his admission. He indulged in many violent acts while under the influence of delusions. Physically, he was running down rapidly, so that it became necessary to restrict his tendency to over-exercise. At this time he claimed that he was "king of gods", that he made all the people of the earth, and that he could raise all who had been dead over fifty years. He claimed that he owned the whole world; that his clothes were covered with diamonds. He wrote and sent off continually telegraphic messages to imaginary persons. He declared that Queen Victoria, the Empress Elizabeth, and the "queen of poets" belonged to him as wives, and that he made them. The patient was very forgetful of common and ordinary names. During the second night of his stay with us the patient thought that he made a trip to Heaven. and gave to one of his friends there one hundred billions of dollars. In the morning he wanted two hundred and fifty millions of gold with which to line his room. He afterward thought that this wish had been complied with. He slept very little for several nights, but after a time greatly improved in this respect. Physically, the patient was very weak and scarcely able to walk, though he imagined that his strength was limitless. His pulse for sometime ranged from 64 to 100. When the pulse was low he seemed much prostrated and enfeebled; when it was high he became wild and incoherent. The pupils varied, the left being generally more dilated than the right. When the left was normal, the right would become contracted. The patient's speech was thick and his words could scarcely be distinguished, yet his delusions were uttely marvellous. At times he would create several worlds in a single night. Again, he would be the possessor of numerous wives and children.

About one month after admission the patient's ideas of wealth passed away. He said that they were only visions, and that he again felt poor. For about two months he gained gradually, both in mind and body. He gave up his delusions and talked rationally, and the only apparent abnormal symptom was a slight tremulousness of lips and tongue when speaking. The patient was discharged at the request of his friends. Although, to the untrained observer, he appeared quite well, the result of his case was entered upon our books as "improved", and his relatives, when pressing us for an opinion as to his future, were assured that he would, in all probability, suffer a relapse within six months, and that he would never fully recover. The sequel proved that our prognosis was correct, for about five months from the date of his discharge the patient was readmitted. It was stated that he had been quiet most of the time during his absence from the hospital, and had attended meetings and gatherings for amusement, but had worked at his business scarcely at all. His friends said that he had generally appeared well, but not always "exactly right". The night before he was returned he became violent, and attempted to kill his wife with a hatchet. He had delusions that enemies were after him, and that he must fight them. He had no apparent ideas of grandeur, and had cherished none during his vacation. A month later the patient had several slight temporary attacks of left-sided paralysis, after which he gradually failed in memory until he did not know his own room. Then he became very wealthy again, and thought that he owned the hospital, and was planning to stock it with millions of dollars worth of goods. He claimed that he had seventy immense and costly stores filled with innumerable goods in New York City. While cherishing these delusions he seemed for a time to improve physically. After a while blisters and sores appeared upon his hands, and then he became less excited and more moderate in his ideas. The ulcers on his hands finally healed, and the patient appeared better mentally, having given up his delusions of wealth. Under ophthalmoscopic examination, atrophy of both discs was revealed. A month later he suffered another attack of temporary paralysis of the left side, and his delusions of wealth revived. He began to steal all the books he could find, and locked them up in his bureau. He was also caught masturbating, although he had heretofore manifested no tendency in that direction. He continued in this condition for about two months, and then gave up his delusions of wealth, and was again depressed. His appetite failed, and he subsisted mainly upon milk and beef tea. Finally, the sphincters became relaxed, and he frequently wet the bed. Two months later he had epileptiform seizures, but rallied from them. He was greatly emaciated, weighing only eighty-two pounds, and yet for a time he appeared once more to be gaining. His appetite improved and his spirits were remarkably exuberant for an almost dead man. The week following he had another epileptiform seizure; it was one of general and severe convulsion. The next day he rallied and could talk, and still he manifested delusions of wealth. He gradually lost in flesh until he weighed but seventy-three and a half pounds. His urine was retained, and it was drawn with a catheter. The patient was unable to swallow, and was fed regularly with a soft rubber nasal tube. A month later the patient passed into a comatose condition from which he rallied, recognized those about him, spoke pleasantly, and assured us that he felt "fuss-rate". A few hours later he quietly died.

A post mortem examination was made, and the scalp was found to be very thin, as was also the skull. On removing the skull-cap, three ounces of serum escaped from the subdural space. The subarachnoid spaces were likewise found to be filled with serum. The arachnoid membrane was decidedly opaque. The pia mater was adherent to the cortical substance of the brain, the result of long continued inflammation. The brain weighed forty-three and three-fourths ounces.

This case presents the most salient points of paresis. The age, forty-one, the very prime of life; the condition, married, but having no children, consequently no bar or interruption to sexual excess; the apparent cause, intemperance, and the final result, death after such marked improvement as to insure the patient's discharge for several months from the hospital; and through a period of nearly two years the persistent abnormality of articulation, and the condition of the pupils, together with the rise and fall of delusions of grandeur and wealth, all these form an imposing array of important and interesting facts.

Mrs. F. E. E., æt. 31. The causes of insanity were put down as "grief and physical debility". At the time of admission this patient was weak and unsteady on her feet. There was slight tremor of the tongue, and on extending the arms and hands, the fingers trembled and twitched constantly. She had a "happy-go-lucky" disposition at times, and again was depressed. She rambled from one subject to another, and took but little interest in her surroundings. Her temperature fluctuated between 99° and 101° F. She had a good appetite, slept well, and appeared perfectly contented, always answering that she felt "first rate" when questioned as to her feelings. Two months from the date of admission the husband removed the patient to her home, but was obliged to return her to the institution seven months later. She was then debilitated, filthy, demented, and inclined to be violent when annoyed. She presented no symptoms of delusions or hallucinations. One using her arms and legs, she exhibited considerable unsteadiness and loss of power. The tongue was very tremulous, and she experienced much trouble in pronouncing certain words. The intellect gradually became weaker and weaker; she omitted words when speaking, and often repeated others several times. She crammed her mouth in an imbecile manner when eating, and had to be watched carefully, to prevent choking. The patient gradually became more helpless and demented, dazed and feeble. There were sordes on the teeth, the tongue was red, and pointed to the left side. The skin bruised easily, and was cold and dry, flaking off easily. Later the patient was unable to swallow solid food. The body became covered with red spots, and the temperature rose to 102.2° F. The eruption disappeared quickly, and the temperature fell to normal. At this time the patient was in a condition of absolute dementia, with muscular atrophy throughout the entire body; and legs, arms and hands were contracted. About two weeks later she passed away.

Here was a case demented almost from the very first, and at no time presenting any delusions of grandeur, wealth or position; and although the patient was practically bedridden from the inception of the disease, she lived over four years.

Causes

We come now to consider some of the causes of general paresis.

A nervo-sanguine temperament, great physical activity, vaulting ambition, imperfect education (many men go into fields of great enterprises with very limited education, and with only half-trained brains), a desire to attain and enjoy all good things in life, coupled with anxiety and worry—that is, fear lest the object in view may not be gained, or if gained, may be unsatisfactory—these are the substrata of conditions upon which the superstructure of general paresis almost always rests.

The paretic is an adventurer, an explorer, a discoverer of new means for the acquirement of wealth, a diviner with a magic wand of imagination that conjures up golden Golcondas in every business scheme. Some of the most brilliant toilers and workers for the growth of this new land have finally succumbed to paresis. Some of the brainiest of actors, and wittiest of writers, and most zealous of politicians, and skilful managers of great railroad systems, have yielded to this dire disease; and the cause lies in a hyperstimulation of the brain and nervous system by such means as hard work, coupled with hard drinking, excessive sexual indulgence, and an all-absorbing worry about every undertaking, whether it be in the world of business or in the field of pleasure.

Clouston says that "the things that most excite and at the same time most exhaust the highest brain energy are those which tend most strongly to cause the disease; to wit, over and promiscuous sexual indulgence combined with hard muscular labor, a stimulating diet of highly-fed flesh meat, the being all the while excited and poisoned by alcohol and syphilis; all these things begun early in life and kept as steadily." He declares that in Scotland "the Durham miner when earning good wages fulfils the most perfect conditions for the production of general paralysis. Every sixth lunatic admitted to the Durham County Asylum is a general paralytic." Clouston also states that "the Asiatic is not subject to paresis, that the savage is free from it, and that the Irishman and Scotch Highlander must go to the big towns or to America to have the distinction of being able to acquire it." There are comparatively few cases of general paresis where the causes may not be traced to overwork in the field of worry, wine and women. Some European authors have claimed that every case of paresis is tainted with syphilis. While it is true that paretics are likely to be exposed to syphilitic infection, it is not, we believe, either the universal cause or the invariable accompaniment of paresis. We can hardly accept the dictum of the Austrian professor of syphilitic diseases. After listening to a lecture in Vienna, I asked the professor if he had noticed the effect of syphilis in the production of insanity. He replied that he had not considered the matter, and could not give the desired information, but closed his remarks smilingly by saying: "You know, Doctor, that the whole civilized world is *syphilized!*" We will admit that a considerable portion of the victims of paresis have the syphilitic taint, but there are some paretic patients whose sexual habits have been correct so far as could be ascertained, and who have suffered only with worry and anxiety about business affairs. Such cases have overtaxed their physical and mental powers, and produced inflammatory conditions of the brain; but they have neither tarried too long at the wine cup, nor indulged in promiscuous salacity.

Imperfect education, a bounding ambition, and a feeling that one's strength will never give out may rank as predispositions to paresis. A young man with hopeful disposition, and strong, full-blooded physique, will work and play with such a lack of judgement as to land him at last in the bottomless pit of paresis. Full of hope and health, he does not realize the fact that there is a possibility of breaking down when he works like a slave all day, and enjoys festivities like a Satyr and an Epicure all night.

In considering the causation of paresis, we note the influence of sex, and find that at the Middletown State Homeopathic Hospital there have been thus far under treatment two hundred and fifty male paretics and thirty-one female paretics. Possibly men work harder and worry more than women, and they may be less elastic than those of the opposite sex in meeting and braving the ordinary vicissitudes of life.

Paretics are more numerous in cities and in seaport towns than in the country. It is also a notable fact that most paretics are very fond of rich meats and of strong coffee. A vegetarian mode of living would probably save many from this disease.

Paresis develops usually between the ages of twenty-five and fifty years. Dr. Clouston tells of a case which developed at the age of sixteen, and Dr. Guislain reports one at the age of seventeen. Occasionally this disease may develop in old age, but the insanity of that period of life usually takes on the form of senile dementia, with its many-colored vagaries, instead of paresis.

PATHOLOGY

The inflammations of paresis seem to involve in a general way those portions of the cerebral membranes which cover the frontal and parietal lobes. Dr. Clouston has stated that when the mental symptoms are most severe the inflammatory processes will be found located on the anterior and upper convolutions of the brain. If convulsive tendencies are present, then these inflammatory patches will be found

GENERAL PARESIS

at the base of the brain, and in the region of the fourth ventricle. Also, Broca's convolution is much involved when the speech has been especially affected. The meninges in paresis are usually inflamed and thickened, and the pia mater—that is, the inner membrane—is adherent in small pin point spots to the brain cortex. Under the influence of inflammation and the thickening of the membranes, the brain mass itself becomes compressed, and we have a condition of atrophy of the nerve cells during the latter stage of the disease. It has seemed to me, also, that there has occurred in many cases an hypertrophic metamorphosis of the neuroglia. In other words, the mass of cellular connective tissue which keeps in place the nerve cells and the nerve fibres in the cerebrum has become thickened. When this occurs, there is pressure not only from above downward, but from below upward, and from within outward, thus placing the nerve cells and the nerve wires of communication from the brain to the various parts of the body between what may be termed upper and nether pathological millstones. Sometimes the disease appears to start in the spinal cord and work upward to the brain, and sometimes the disease begins at the top of the brain and works down into the cord.

The pia mater when peeled from the paretic brain takes with it small, fine portions of the cerebral substance. The arachnoid membrane sometimes becomes opaque, and has small flaky deposits, together with serous effusions. The dura mater is commonly thickened and gorged with blood, and it presents a loose, leathery, roughened appearance, which is a strange contrast to the fine, smooth, closely woven condition of the membrane in health. Occasionally tumors of a gummatous nature are found in the brain of paretics. Atrophy and sclerosis of the cerebral mass, and likewise of the great nerve tracks of the body, are conditions generally found. The lungs of the paretic are usually sound, but there is shallow respiration. The heart becomes weak and uncertain in its action; the kidneys are somewhat degenerated, and symptoms of Bright's disease now and then present themselves.

Diagnosis, Prognosis and Treatment

Paresis may be confounded with locomotor ataxia, progressive muscular atrophy, and senile dementia. While the muscular movements may simulate those of ataxia and atrophy, you will remember that mental aberration does not usually accompany locomotor ataxia or muscular atrophy. Senile dementia may be distinguished quite commonly from paresis by the age of the patient, and by the absence of those very exalted delusions which paresis engenders. From alcoholic dementia it may be distinguished by the history of the case, and by careful observation. The alcoholic dement is more vague and uncertain and less persistent in his delusions than the paretic. Of course if a drunkard and a paretic are locked up in a hospital and kept under observation for a sufficient length of time, the drunkard will get well, while the paretic will continue on his pathological toboggan slide to the end.

The prognosis is unfavourable, and usually the patient dies within from one to eight or ten years after the inception of the disease. By means of rest in bed, and a suitable diet, and proper care, the paretic may live for several years. Whether the patient is in bed, or up and dressed, he should be afforded an abundance of fresh air and balmy sunshine. These blessings should be brought to him; he should not be obliged to run after them. He should also be protected from severe draughts of cold air, as the skin is apt to be

GENERAL PARESIS

flabby and moist, with a sticky perspiration, and consequently he may easily take cold. On the other hand, he should be protected from the rays of a hot sun, because excessive heat is extremely prostrating and injurious to the average paretic patient.

Paretic patients should be secluded from every care and toil. During remissions they may exercise very gently, but they should be kept in bed when they have reached the weak and tottering stage. They should not be allowed to associate with other excited patients, or run any risk of getting bruised or tumbled about.

The beds for paretic patients should be soft, elastic, and comfortable in every particular, to avoid, so far as possible, the danger of bed-sores. The patient's skin should be kept clean and firm by the use of alcohol baths, applied with a sponge, about once in forty-eight hours; and wherever pressure occurs the skin should be oiled once or twice a day with coconut oil, gently but carefully rubbed in. By a judicious use of oil, and alcohol and water, and by the use of proper beds, and by skilful nursing, the paretic patient will avoid, as far as possible, the distressing annoyance of that *bête noire* of the hospital—namely, the bed-sore. If, in spite of every precaution, a bed-sore should occur, then it may be cleansed with Calendula tincture diluted with water, three parts of the former to one hundred parts of the latter. The ulcer may then be packed with Bichloride of Murcury, one to five thousand. Should the process of suppuration make deep inroads, then Peroxide of Hydrogen will cleanse and help to heal all the byways where pus is inclined to form and pocket. Vaseline with Calendula or Carbolic Acid may be applied as an emollient dressing, after the ulcer has been thoroughly cleansed. A smooth bed and scrupulous cleanliness are the main essentials in the treatment of a bed-sore.

If you are called upon to select a climate for a paretic, you should recommend Florida or Southern California during the winter, and a slow, easy march to the North when hot weather comes on. But if the patient is unable to travel, then a moderate and uniform climate should be selected if possible. If you cannot regulate the climate, then you should regulate the temperature of the room in which the patient is kept, and if you can maintain it at from 68 to 70 degrees Fahrenheit, you will do what is best for your patient.

Prevention

The question now arises: What shall be done to save men and women from the inception and invasion of this fell scourge? For fifty years the task of curing general paresis has been attempted by faithful and learned men, yet with only negative or unsuccessful results. While we may record with pride a series of triumphs against the ordinary foes of life, we stand aghast before the inroads of this unyelding vampire. Such being the fact, would it not be wise to apply the means for prevention, rather than engage in the discouraging task of patching up or seeking to save the shattered fragments of an inevitable wreck? The causes of paresis have been pointed out. Prominent among these figure worriments, and intemperance of various kinds. To prevent the growth and development of these subtle causes among the young, the vigorous and the successful, we must give to them a better education, a loftier purpose to shun evil and to do right, a clearer knowledge of what that right is, and a most invincible determination to accomplish the greatest good in life without shattering one's forces upon the rocks of dangerous and needless excess. When the people, through advice and warning from their physicians, are brought to know and to realize the fatality of their own self-imposed diseases, they may then, perhaps, be induced to refrain from those formidable dissipations whose feet take hold on destruction, whose bite is like that of an adder, and whose final resting place is a hopeless chamber and a death-bed within the walls of a hospital for the insane.

The cares and afflictions of ordinary life, the reverses of fortune, the depletions of disease, the hereditary weaknesses which come down to us from our ancestors, all bring to institutions for the insane their quota of suffering victims; but many who are thus afflicted may be stimulated by the hope of restoration, and may indeed get well and return in due time to their homes, and to a life of usefulness. But for him who progresses to paresis through the devious ways of his own worriments, and dissipations, and gorgings, and exhaustions, there are no more cheering words than those engraved upon the portals of Dante's Inferno:

"Who enters here, leaves hope behind."

Young gentlemen: We have led you over a long and tedious pathway. The march has been dry and dusty, yet you have borne the heat and burden of the day with a patient fortitude. I trust that you have come to realize the importance of learning something about insanity. It is imperative that you, as progressive physicians, should know something of insanity, because it is prevalent everywhere, among all classes and grades of people—the mighty and the lowly, the poor and the rich. Again, you should know something about its modern treatment. It is a difficult disease to treat and to cure, and yet some recoveries are attained by a practical application of the Hospital Idea.

As we study and investigate this question aright, we are forced to the conclusion that insanity is an almost universal disease. It has, indeed, been a most dreaded scourge throughout the ages. As we examine the pages of history, we find that this terrible disorder has stalked through the high places of the palaces of the old Roman Cæsars. It has swept down like a Black Death upon the thrones of Spain, of France, of Austria, and of Italy. It has buried its cruel fangs in the brains of Bavarian and Belgian monarchs. It has moved upon Russia with a force greater than that which accompanied Napoleon when he marched through snow and ice upon the burning city of Moscow. It has sat at meat with the mightiest rulers of Great Britain, converting them into maniacs and dements, whose presence upon the throne has formed the darkest blot upon the pages of English history. And it has traversed the mountains of the North, and infested that fair and favoured land which was once blest with the rulership of a Gustavus Adolphus, and inspired by the songs of a Jenny Lind.

Prince, peasant, and pauper alike have felt the blighting touch of this withering witch who has spread her death-wand over the civilized world for many centuries, and whose ravishing activity is today sapping the vitality and dissipating the mental energy of the strongest nations on earth.

It is our duty to disclose the nature and the dangers of insanity, and it is your duty to learn something about it, in order that you may be able to assist in its prevention, and in its appropriate treatment. No one-sided philosophy will explain its nature, and no routine practice dispel her enchantment. Only the earnest student who studies this aberration of mind without fear and without prejudice will learn the secret of its enchantment, and so dissolve the spell.

Who shall cure this dread disease? Only the patient psychologist, the enthusiastic student, the philosophical physician, and the earnest and zealous philanthropist. The task is a mighty one, and in its accomplishment one needs the courage of the soldier, the zeal of the preacher, and the heroism of him who would recue from midnight flames the helpless victim of a conflagration. He who engages in this work of leading the insane back to health, and who spares no measure of brain or blood in the act, is a person who is deserving of that glorious epitaph of Lamartine's: "Workman in the cause of humanity."

Lecture IX

TREATMENT

We now approach the last, yet most important division of our subject,—namely, the Treatment of the Insane.

When you are called to see a case of insanity, you may be required to decide upon the disposition of the case. That is, you may have to determine as to whether the patient shall remain at home, or go to a private sanitarium, or be committed to a State hospital for the insane.

In all ages, the disease known as insanity has been regarded as a disgrace, more or less, hence it has been concealed from general observation both by the patient and his friends. This concealment of mental weakness or aberration is natural, because the human being is so constructed that he almost always endeavours to hide his defects of both body and mind. Therefore, when you are called to treat a case of insanity, you should not hastily consign the victim to a public hospital, for by so doing you may put a public stamp upon the entire subsequent life of your patient. That a person has been insane should not be regarded a disgrace, but simply a misfortune; yet the fact remains that when once his insanity is known, the person is always afterward likely to be regarded with suspicion and distrust by those around him. That feeling will by and by, in the coming enlightenment of the world, pass away, but until it does we must consider its effect in the disposition of each case brought to our attention.

Home Treatment.—Some insane patients may be cared for at home, although, as a general rule, the disagreements with home life, experienced by the insane man, are a bar to recovery. Home treatment may, however, be attempted for the following class of cases:

1. Those who are wealthy, and who can afford the luxury of every possible care. Such patients may be put in charge of trained nurses and experienced physicians, if the friends are willing to convert a portion of the house into a hospital, and are willing to refrain from interfering with the necessary care and treatment. If the attending physician cannot control and direct the treatment absolutely at home, then he should suggest a change.

2. Quiet and harmless insane patients—that is, cases of chronic melancholia where the delusions have crystallized, and where the disposition to suicide has subsided. Also, there are cases of chronic dementia, or of imbecility, or of senile dementia, that may be cared for in private homes or in cottages, if a reasonable amount of patience and tact and watchfulness can be exercised in their behalf. In treating the insane, you should always consider, first, the feasibility of home treatment.

Sanitariums.—When the interests of the patient, or the highest interests of the friends demand that the insane person should be removed from home, then the next question to decide is: Where shall he go? If he is blest with the luxury of wealth, he may be sent to a sanitarium, if a suitable one can be discovered. Great care should be used in the selection of a sanitarium. The welfare of the patient will depend upon the nature and character of the man in charge of such a place. If the spirit of advice holds sway, then it is likely that the patient will get but small return for a large outlay. Private sanitariums should be carefully inspected by public officials in such a way as to promote the interests of the patients, and in such a manner as to accomplish fair and just results between man and man. Sanitariums have their advantages. By going to such a place the insane man is enabled, oftentimes, to hide his disease, and consequently his fancied disgrace, from his neighbours. If he can go to a sanitarium and get well, he returns to his home and the community where he formerly lived, and immediately takes his old place in good and regular standing. He has simply been absent from home, to recuperate from nervous prostration.

State Hospitals.—When the resources of the home and of the sanitarium have failed, or when the financial ability of the patient can no longer meet the strain of either home or sanitarium care, then a public hospital that is free to the poor, and moderate in its charges to those who have a little money left, may be secured. To this end, the State hospitals have been established.

When a patient is sent to a State hospital the method should be straightforward and honest. If able to comprehend anything, he should be frankly told that he is suffering from mental disturbance, and that his friends propose taking him to an institution for treatment. He may object, but his scruples may often be overcome by kindly reasoning. If that is of no avail, then force, rather than deception, should be resorted to. Everything pertaining to his removal should be conducted in a prompt and orderly manner after a preconceived plan.

Treatment

The means which we have employed at Middletown for treating the insane may be put down as follows:

1. Kindness and gentle discipline.
2. Rest as a means of physical and mental recuperation.
3. Bathing and massage.
4. Enforced protection.

5. Artificial feeding.
6. Dietetics.
7. Exercise, amusement and occupation.
8. Moral hygiene.
9. Medicine.

Kindness and Gentle Discipline.—Formerly insanity was considered as a visitation from the Devil, a possession in every fibre by his Satanic Majesty, and the treatment consisted of punishment—such punishment as confinement in a dark cell for the comfort of the soul, chains for the aching limbs, stripes for the back, shower baths for the heated blood, and for the drooping heart there were conjured up the inspiring influences of gaunt and ghastly fear! But, today, the treatment of the insane is based upon the broad and comprehensive principle which is embodied and shadowed forth in the precepts of the Golden Rule. Kindness is the Blarney Stone which every man, who would attempt the work of treating disordered intellects. must kiss, and thus imbibe its inspiration. To be sure, the insane must be controlled and governed, but while the administration of discipline is at times necessarily firm and unyielding, it should in every word and action be tinctured with the essence of human benevolence. The more irresponsible the patient, the gentler and more sympathetic should be the treatment. As patients resume their normal condition, they may be more and more subjected to the influence of laws necessary for proper government. As loss of self-control is a prominent indication of insanity, so a resumption of self-restraint is a pleasant indication of approaching recovery.

Rest in Bed.—When a patient is admitted the hospital he is at once carefully examined by one of the medical officers of the institution, and if he seems debilitated, even though manifestaing much excitement and insane strength, he is sent to one of the hospital wards and placed in bed, where he may be under the constant care of trained and skilled nurses. For many years we have made constant repose in comfortable beds a prime adjuvant in the treatment and cure of insanity, and in prolonging the lives and promoting the comfort of those who are aged and feeble and unlikely to recover. We find that the victims of every form of insanity, whether that form be characterized by mental depression, or mental exaltation, or mental enfeeblement, or mental failure, are greatly benefited by bed treatment. The victims of melancholia rise more surely from the "slough of despond" when placed in bed, and properly nourished and protected from every adverse exposure, than when they are allowed to sit up and be dressed. The victims of mania become quiet and tractable, and make better progress toward recovery in bed than anywhere else. The victims of general paresis are less liable to receive injuries, and their paroxysms of tremulous excitement subside sooner when placed in bed than when they are dressed and staggering about the ward. The victims of dementia are less filthy, and can be better cared for and made more comfortable in every way when in bed than when up and dressed, and planted in chairs along the corridors of hospital wards. Apathetic and depressed patients are not only less filthy when subjected to careful hospital treatment in bed than when up and around the ward, but they also sleep more during the twenty-four hours than they otherwise would. They likewise take their food better, and thus physically thrive more prosperously than when out of bed. We have observed many cases where patients on being taken from the bed and dressed would refuse to eat their food, but when returned to a recumbent position upon an easy mattress they would immediately begin to take their customary rations.

The advantages of this plan are:

1. The waning forces of the patients are most surely conserved.

2. An easy circulation of the blood throughout the entire system is facilitated, and thus the wastes produced by disease are most speedily and naturally repaired.

3. Digestion and assimilation of suitable food, in cases where the normal functions of the body are much below par, are best promoted in bed, providing suitable care and treatment are administered.

4. The patients are more readily protected from injuries when in bed than when dressed and allowed to wander about the ward in association with disturbed or violent patients.

5. The application of heat is most readily made, and its benefits most uniformly secured when the patients are in bed and carefully covered with suitable clothing. The danger of exposing the extremities to chilling draughts is thus most surely averted.

6. Attendants treat bed patients with more tender consideration than they usually bestow upon cases that are dressed and move about the ward. A sick person when in bed always excites more kindly sympathy and more attentive care than when he is attired in his usual clothing, and moving about among his fellows.

7. An insane person if weak in body, and either excited or depressed or apathetic in mind, recovers more rapidly and certainly when afforded proper bed treatment than when allowed the freedom of daily exercise. I believe that many of the insane may be saved from the trackless realms of chronic dementia if suitable rest treatment is afforded

and enforced during the stormy, or sullen, or obfuscated experiences of mania, or melancholia, or acute dementia.

Rest in bed does not mean neglect by nurses. On the contrary, it means increased care by specially trained nurses. The patient must be carefully and regularly looked after; his skin must be kept in good condition; his mouth must be cleansed with pure water at regular intervals; the bowels, if constipated must be relieved by enemas of warm water; the bladder must be emptied of its contents as often as that organ becomes filled; and baths of various kinds must be given.

We use baths as follows:

1. The simple towel or sponge bath, where the patient's body is laved a little at a time with alcohol and water—one part of alcohol to four or five parts of water,—and then the part is rubbed until dry.

2. The spray bath is used for those who are strong enough to sit up. This bath not only cleanses the skin, but stimulates by its fine and exhilarating force the subcutaneous nerves throughout the system.

3. The old-fashioned tub bath is given to those who desire it, using warm water at the outset, and finishing with cold water and a brisk rubbing.

Bed patients also receive massage when necessary, and they are sometimes anointed, from head to foot, every night with coconut oil, or olive oil. We use, externally, when the patient seems very much strained and exhausted, cocoanut oil, ninetyfive parts, and Hypericum tincture, five parts. Hypericum is called, as you know, the "Arnica of the nerves", and this preparation is a most stoothing and agreeable one. If the patient has, upon admission, recent bruises upon the body, we apply Arnica and oil in the same way.

Old bruises which are dark from subcutaneous hemorrhages may be treated with Hamamelis and oil.

Enforced Protection.—Many of the weak and exhausted patients coming to us for treatment are quite willing to rest in bed. They are already the victims of overwork, and rest comes to them as a boon which has been desired for years, but which could not heretofore be attained. Others require to be restrained to a certain extent. This restraint, or care, or protection may be applied by a nurse who will put the patient back to bed whenever he gets up, and kindly encourage him to remain there; or, if that is insufficient, we use a body bandage. That is, a band is placed around the waist and fastened at the back with soft tapes. On either side of the body bandage is a strip of cloth that is tied around the bed rail. The restless, incoherent, and harmless patient is kept quiet by this means, for he finds, after a little, that he cannot get up, and therefore stops trying to do so. Others are restless all over; constantly moving the legs, the arms, the body, and the head. In such cases we apply what is known as the "protection sheet", which is an addition to the body bandage, and which covers the entire body, with the exception of the head and neck. When this protection sheet is carefully applied, the patient cannot get out of bed, nor can he hurt himself in any way. If his knees are chafed from motion, then he should wear drawers, or a bandage may be applied, extending from the ankle to the middle of the thigh. An ordinary surgical bandage applied as if to hold a splint in place will answer the purpose.

Some patients are pugilistic, and inclined to hurt others; or they are suicidal, and inclined to mutilate themselves. We protect such cases by the use of padded mittens. Large canvas mittens are made and padded with cotton, and inside the cotton we place a smaller mitten to hold the hand. When these mittens are properly used, the patient can do but little damage to either himself or others. (The "protection sheet" was first applied at the Middletown State Hospital over eighteen years ago, and it has been used here, as needed, ever since. It has also been introduced into many of the progressive institutions of this country.)

In your private practice, you may be called upon suddenly to take care of a very violent and restless case, and if you have no appliances at hand, you may make a cocoon by taking three or four common sheets, such as you will find in every house. Sew these together, and roll them up like an ordinary bandage, and then apply the bandage to the entire body, from the head down, just as you would bandage an arm or a leg. You may pinion the arms to the sides of the body, before applying the cocoon, with long towels or strips of cloth. When a patient is rolled up in the cocoon, and the end of the roll is fastened with safety pins, you may put him in bed, and he cannot get out, or move around at all. The cocoon is simple and effective. If you are obliged to apply the cocoon rather snugly, as in the case of a fiercely excited patient, it is wise to put a few layers of cotton over the chest, to relieve the inflexbiliity of the bandage.

Exercise, Amusement and Occupation.—After the newly admitted patients have been favored with rest treatment for a sufficient length of time (and that time may be one month, or three months, or six months, or twelve months), then we prescribe exercise, amusement, and occupation for them. At first they are allowed to sit up in an easy chair; then they are allowed to walk around the day-rooms, then they are permitted to play on the piano, or play cards, or dominoes, or billiards. A little later they are allowed to exercise on the grounds. The exercise is increased until the patients are sufficiently hardened to engage in some useful occupation, such as working to engage in some useful occupation, such as working on the wards, or in the dining-rooms, or in the sewing-rooms, or folding clothes in the laundry, or cultivating flowers in the greenhouse, or promoting the growth of vegetables and grains in the garden on the farm. By such a course of treatment we have had the pleasure of seeing apparently hopeless cases, after long periods of rest and nourishment, rise from sick beds and progress to genuine and substantial recoveries. After rest and care and nourishment have effected both physical and mental recuperation, then the duties and burdens of life may be gradually reassumed. But labor should be imposed in very moderate doses, and the drug of toil should be given in the attenuated form.

In the care and treatment of the insane great caution should be exercised while the almost recovered are completing the term of convalescence. As the twilight and the dawn are the most dangerous seasons for those of suicidal tendencies, so the last days of convalescence, when the patient is feeling once more the impulses of recovery, are oftentimes critical periods which need special attention.

Artificial Feeding.—Insanity is a symptom not only of mental aberration, but likewise of physical depletion and cerebral exhaustion. Especially is this true with regard to the various forms, shades and degrees of melancholia and mania. We find in those suffering with mental depression, oftentimes a direct lack of desire for food, while those laboring under a stress of mental exaltation are quite apt to neglect the inception of nourishment through inattention rather than through anorexia.

The first essential in the dietetic treatment of the unwilling insane for curative purposes is the enforced administration of sufficient quantities of food, to prevent too rapid waste throughout the individual system, and to promote recuperation from losses already sustained; and likewise to increase, if possible, the capitalized resources of the human form divine.

The second essential is the selection of such food as will most rapidly and surely promote the rebuilding of those portions of the human temple which have been disgruntled or shattered by the effects of disease.

The third essential is the administration of the selected food in such a manner as to avoid all unnecessary shocks; to promote, in fact, easy and rapid digestion, and to favor the speedy assimilation of digested food by the tissues of the body. In our experience we have found that forced feeding may most readily be applied by the use of a soft rubber naso-stomach tube. This tube, as now used, was the invention of one of my former assistants, Dr. N. Emmons Paine, and is a modification, both in constructions and use, of the soft rubber catheter of Nélation. When this tube has been inserted through the nose, and passed on to the stomach, by a physician or skilled nurse, the food may be injected through it in required quantities by means of an ordinary rubber syringe.

Those who continue the administration of food through the old-fashioned stomach tube prefer, as a rule, I believe, that the patient shall be in a sitting posture when fed; but when using Dr. Paine's soft rubber naso-stomach tube it seems preferable to have the patient lying on his back. In this supine position, the patient is less able to voluntarily regurgitate his food than when he is allowed to sit up. This is an important clinical fact, because many patients who need forced feeding are apt to acquire the habit of regurgitating food when they are thus fed. This they can do less easily when in a supine position than when sitting upright.

Now in addition to the method of forced feedings, to which we have referred, we may state that in feeding indifferent and unwilling insane patients it is always wise to begin by coaxing and persuading the sick person in the gentlest and most tactful manner to accept food voluntarily rather than to have it forced into his stomach. Many a reluctant patient will eat when properly and persistently coaxed by a skilful and judicious nurse.

Dietetics.—We come now to a consideration of the varieties of food best adapted to those depletions and exhaustions which precede and accompany mental and nervous diseases.

Owing to the restlessness and the exhaustion of the insane and to the fact that the life forces wane rapidly, and the blood inclines to lose some of its natural fluidity, it seems to me that the diet at the outset should consist largely of hot liquid foods, and principally of milk. The disrepute into which milk has sometimes fallen as an article of diet for either the sick or the well has arisen from the fact, to a large extent, I believe, that it has been administered cold instead of warm. Coming from the ice chest, or sipped from a glass filled with lumps of impure and death-dealing ice, and after being taken from diseased cows, it has often been a dangerous diet for even the most healthy. When milk is taken cold in large quantities it chills the weak stomach of the invalid; it curdles and forms indigestible lumps; and it ferments and brews putrescent gases in the intestines. But when pure milk is brought to a blood heat, or a higher temperature than blood, and then administered to the worn and exhausted victim of disease, it favors digestion and assimilation and prevents, to a very large extent, the evils of cold milk to which we have referred. If you have any doubt as to the purity of the milk you use, you should have it sterilized. This can be done in any house by putting the milk in a clean vessel, and bringing it up to heat of 160°F., and keeping it there about twenty minutes. This process destroys the germs without seriously changing the quality of the milk. You should always procure milk which has been cleansed by the use of a separator.

In addition to milk, you may give beef tea, bean broth, and chicken, clam, oyster, and other soups. You may also give gruels made of oats, and barley, and wheat, and rice, and corn, and other cereals. You may give soups containing much cream, and flavored with such vegetables as celery, and lettuce, and tomato, and beans or peas; and you will find the various concentrated foods valuable aids to treatment.

An exhausted invalid should take food in moderate quantities, in order to avoid overtaxing the powers of a weakened stomach, and after each ingestion of food the organs of digestion should be allowed to do their work fully, after which a brief period of rest may be enjoyed. But this rest should not be long continued, for if it is, then exhaustion of the patient, through lack of proper and necessary nutrition, speedily follows.

After many experiments, we have concluded that a weak insane person should be fed once every three hours, from 6 A.M. till 9 P.M. and if the patient is sleepless during the night, then the food may be continued every three hours throughout the entire day and night.

Hot milk may, with almost absolute safety, form the daily diet and the midnight hypnotic of the mental invalid. Should such a food prove too rich in some individual case, then the milk may be diluted with lime water, or with clysmic, or seltzer water. Should the proportion of cream in milk seem too large, then it may be reduced by skimming. Thus the amount of fat to be administered to a given patient may be regulated, by experience to meet the actual necessities of the case. You may also enrich milk by the addition of cream when necessary for the better nourishment of emaciated cases. The cream diet may be improved by whipping up the white of an egg with about four times its bulk of cream.

Aged patients are often benefited by the use of buttermilk. In fact, all patients who have easily disordered kidneys may be almost invariably benefited by the use of fresh buttermilk.

If you have a patient who is very fat and flabby, or who is suffering with dyspepsia, you may begin the rest treatment with skimmed milk for two or three weeks, in order to allow the useless débris to pass away from the system.

While a hot liquid diet is being administered the patient may, if he craves solid food, be treated two or three times a day to a slice of of toasted stale bread of such variety as he may select—that is, either white bread, or graham bread, or rye bread.

After a patient has, by the use of a hot liquid diet, fleshed somewhat beyond his normal weight, then he may be allowed solid food, consisting largely of the various native and imported grains, together with vegetables and fruits, and a very moderate supply of meat. Rich and stimulating red meat is sometimes good for cases of melancholia, but cases of mania and general paresis should be restricted as to the eating of meat. It sometimes stimulates too much those who are excitable and nervous. Meat should also be withheld from those who are suffering with epileptic insanity. During convalescence, patients may take a good deal of fat-producing food with benefit. It is better for the nervous and the excitable to take, instead of much meat, plenty of butter, and salad oil, and cod-liver oil. It is always a good plan to get the patient fat as quickly as possible, but while undergoing the process, a sufficient amount of mental stimulus must be applied to keep the brain in moderately active working order while the bodily recuperation is going on. Thus the danger of dementia is averted to a considerable extent.

With the grain foods there may be given an abundance of fresh butter and ripened cheese, or both. Butter and cheese are simply the concentrated products of milk, and they are therefore to be reckoned among the best articles of nutrition for the human body.

Raw or rare cooked eggs go well with milk; and fat bacon or fat spring lamb, with baked potatoes, form excellent additions to the dietary used for the permanent recovery of the convalescent insane. Fruit is allowable in abundant quantities during convalescence. It is said that the ancients when they felt the approaches of old age went down into the gardens of Hesperides and ate apples in large quantities, and thus renewed their youth.

By such a primary and secondary, or combined course of dietetics, the nervous systems of mental invalids are "renewed like the eagle's"; and also by the administration of a moderate daily exercise, in conjunction with solid diet, the muscle tissues become strong again, and ready for active use in the customary walks of life.

Above all things the quality of the food given to the insane should be of the best, and its preparation for consumption should be made with the anxious care of a mother, the delicate tact of a sister, and the scientific skill of an accomplished *chef*. Those who prepare food for the use of human beings should be earnest students of psychological effects, as well as adepts in the esthetics of cookery. The attainment of desired results in the preparation and administration of food for and to both the sick and the well is a lofty and growing ideal, and worthy of the careful study and the critical attention of every one who is interested in the prolongation of human life, and in the preservation and continuance of health. And the food, after it has been prepared as attractively as possible, should be served with dainty delicacy. The refined air and the scrupulous neatness of a restaurant kept by a Delmonico should be assumed in the wards of every hospital, even when only a glass of milk is being served to an insane patient.

Every insane person should have at all times free access to fresh water for drinking purposes. Some persons who avoid fresh water while in their right minds will drink plenty of it when they are insane, and it seems to do them a great deal of good.

Stimulants are rarely needed for those suffering with insanity. The brain is in a hypersensitive condition in such cases, and cannot well endure the added irritation which comes from the use of alcoholic liquors. Yet there are cases of great debility, where the stomach is too weak to retain and digest food, where champagne in small doses may be administered with beneficial effects. Sometimes brandy or whisky may be needed to stimulate the flagging energies of a weak and failing heart. But such a resource is an infrequent necessity. When stimulants are given, only the best and purest articles should be employed.

Moral Hygiene.—Moral hygiene is just as essential in the treatment of insane persons as food is necessary for the mitigation of hunger. Moral hygiene consists in transmitting soul encouragement from the strong to the weak. Doctors and nurses should seek by kind and soothing and stirring words to inspire new spiritual energy in the lives and motives of their patients. Many a patient has been erratic and undisciplined throughout his life, and it is this lack of discipline which often brings a patient to a hospital for the insane. The establishment of mild but judicious direction on the part of those in charge of such patients is a prominent portion of their duty. Every faculty must be cultivated by means of moral hygiene; every emotion must be restrained, and every passion must be subdued, in order to enable mental invalids to possess that perfect self-control which is the loftiest attribute of sanity and strength. The gift of administering moral hygiene is sometimes a natural one, but even natural gifts may be cultivated and strengthened. Hence it is the duty of the physician and the nurse to understand one's self, to cultivate one's own powers, to be inspired by noble purposes, so that the work of transmitting inspirations and disciplinary measures may be successful. This is the aim of all modern schools of psychology.

OPERATIONS

In the treatment of mental disorders, operations have been made for the relief of epilepsy, and for the relief of traumatic injuries. In some instances pressure upon the brain may be relieved, but a cure does not often follow an operation where epilepsy has become firmly established.

It is thought by some that orificial surgery will accomplish much for the insane. Operations for the relief of disorders of the distal extremities of the digestive apparatus have been performed in numerous instances, and these operations, it is said, have resulted in beneficial effects not only to the local physical disorders, but likewise to the general nervous system. Our own experience in these matters has been limited. We have relied not so much upon an operation as upon position, rest, and absolute cleanliness. Rectal diseases are often much relieved by prolonged rest in bed, thus relieving pressure upon all of the pelvic organs. Hot water, both external and internal, aids in relieving chronic congestions and constipations. The homeopathic remedy, appropriately applied, will do its work most thoroughly and satisfactorily, when the patient is in bed, and suitably cared for by a trained nurse. We had one case where the orificial operation was not successful, and through disappointment the patient became a victim of melancholy. This case was put to bed, and the large ulcers around the remnants of his rectum were successfully healed, and the patient regained his normal mental status.

We have also had under our notice cases of insanity in women who have had a part or all of the reproductive organs removed by the surgeon. In some instances it has seemed that the disease preceding the operation has tended to mental disturbance, while in other instances the insanity has followed the operation as an apparent result of shock, hemorrhage, and radically changed physical condition within the human temple.

I believe that a careful discrimination should be exercised by the surgeon in the performance of every capital operation, and that the possibility of mental disorder following a severe operation should be weighed before the undertaking is consummated. It has been demonstrated that formidable operations may be performed without much loss of life, but if the last state of a diseased victim is to be worse than the first, as the result of a grave operation, then it seems to me that the wiser course would be to refrain from using the knife in such a case. It is possible for a woman to live in comparative comfort, and with a good deal of serenity of mind for many years even when afflicted with organic disease of the reproductive system, by the adoption of appropriate hygienic and dietetic measures, and by scientific medication. The simple prolongation of life is not the highest aim of the physician or surgeon, especially if it is accompanied with great mental distress. It is better to have one year of peaceful and contented and healthful mind, than it is to have five years of a new life with an added burden of an agonizing soul torture.

In performing a serious operation, the surgeon should not only consider the probability of extending the life of his victim, but also the probability of casting his victim into the toils of protracted, and, very likely, incurable insanity. Therefore, before making any such operation the surgeon should not only consider the physical strength of his patient, and her ability to endure the process of carving, but he should inquire into the mental antecedents and tendencies of his case, and if mental disorder is likely to supervene upon his work, he should refrain from operating, and seek those mild and less heroic measures for continuing life, and, above all, for preserving mental peace and health of mind.

In concluding this lecture on treatment, we wish to impress upon your mind the fact that the treatment of the insane should always be in accordance with the loftiest principles of the Hospital Idea, which seeks to exemplify everything that can be inspired or suggested by the spirit of kindness or sympathy, and which seeks to embody in the line of practical utility everything that can be acquired in behalf of the sick by intelligent human thought or action. The Hospital Idea embraces all that is known in sanitary science as applied to the protection of human life. It embraces all that is known of dietetics as applied to the restoration of impaired physical energy; and it embraces the education and training of nurses, whose nightly vigils are to supplement the daily visits of the physician. The Hospital Idea is the loftiest embodiment of that mighty and far-reaching rule: "Do unto others as ye would that they should do unto you." The Hospital Idea is a topic as vast as ocean depths, as magnificent as mountain peaks, as enduring as are the experiences of sin and sorrow among men. Its application is the last and grandest work of the philanthropist and a sure forerunner of the millennial dawn. The treatment of mental invalids is being more and more idealized from year to year, and the best methods of the general hospital are steadily coming into vogue in those institutions designed and used for the care and treatment of the insane.

Lecture X

MEDICAL TREATMENT

We come now to consider the medical treatment of insanity. The malady itself has been described in its various forms, and while it is interesting to know all that can be learned concerning disease,—concerning its nature, causes, courses and natural conclusions, the most intensely interesting part of medicine is that which relates to the cure of disease; or, if that is impossible, to the relief and comfort of those who suffer from incurable maladies.

Having considered that part of the treatment which relates to hygiene, to sanitation, to diet, to physical rest and repair, we shall now seek to study the art of applying medicine for the cure or relief of the insane. Hahnemann was exceedingly particular about diet and rest, and the avoidance of all exciting causes of physical and mental disorder. But above and beyond all these, he laid peculiar and emphatic stress upon the curative value of properly selected and carefully administered drugs.

In prescribing a remedy for the cure or relief of insanity, as for any other disease, we have, as comprehensive physicians, to consider:

1. The pathological conditions which exist in the physical structure.

2. The mental aberrations which accompany or follow the physical disturbance; and

3. The totality of symptoms as evolved by a careful study of the history of each individual case.

Again, we find that sometimes a given form of insanity leads to a specific group of remedies.

Whenever you are called upon to treat a case of mental disease, you should make a careful examination—

1. As to the physical condition of the entire system.

2. You should seek to discover all abnormal states of the body which may by any possibility lead to a disturbance of the mind.

3. You should seek to discover the various departures from the normal mental status. (Some patients are very cunning, and will deceive the physician unless he makes a most thorough and persistent investigation of the case.)

4. You should make note of all the symptoms gathered, and having these as a basis for your prescription, you should seek to select the indicated remedy according to the Law of Similars.

Let us now turn our attention to a few remedies for melancholia. It has long been supposed that Aurum Metallicum was a princely remedy for suicidal melancholia. Our experience has not sustained this theory. Aurum has often been prescribed in apparently indicated cases, but usually without good effects. We have a remedy in the Materia Medica which has worked very satisfactorily in cases of restless, resistive, agitated and suicidal melancholia, and that remedy is Arsenicum. The patients that Arsenicum has relieved have been those whose physical condition would naturally suggest the administration of that drug. These patients have been much emaciated, and have had wretched appetites. They present a dry, red, tremulous tongue; they exhibit a shrivelled skin, and a haggard and anxious countenance. They look as if they had suffered the tortures of the damned, and that the fiends of hell were still getting in their fine work. The Arsenicum case is very thirsty, but is easily satisfied with a small quantity. The Arsenicum patient is not only inclined to wear himself out by constant exercise, but he is likewise inclined to kill himself, or, failing in that, he is apt to mutilate the body by chewing the fingers, by pulling out the eyelids, by scratching holes in the face and scalp, and by torturing the flesh generally.

For acute melancholia, where the victim is prostrated by shock, where the grief is intensely profound, where the power of weeping, and thus securing relief, has been abolished, there we find Ignatia Amara the relieving remedy. Probably no drug has produced more comforting results in the realms of sorrow and of loss than the St. Ignatius bean. The Ignatia patient wants to be left alone, and is yet sensitive about what she conceives to be the neglect of her friends. For brooding sorrow, following hard luck or bad news, give Ignatia. For the overmastering effects of good news, which impel some women into the hysteric state, give Coffea. While the Ignatia patient generally broods, she sometimes becomes hysterical, and indulges in temporary fits of laughter. The Natrum Muriaticum patients instead of brooding over their troubles or crying inwardly (Ignatia). bubble and boil and shed tears copiously like the old prince and king over their alleged dead brother, as described in "Huckleberry Finn". The more you attempt to quiet them, the more effusively they weep. If contradicted, they become ill-humored and easily provoked, like Chamomilla and Bryonia. Natrum Muriaticum patients are generally thin and anemic, and have a prematurely old age apprearance. This remedy is often indicated in cases of melancholia following intermittent fever, and when the patients have periodic attacks of violent weeping.

Among the cry baby remedies we have Pulsatilla, Nux Moschata, and Cactus. The Pulsatilla patient weeps easily, but smiles through her tears, and is very changeable. The mental state of Pulsatilla is like the weather in April. Now you see the brilliant radiance of the summer's sun as it glints down from cerulean-hued heavens; and again, you see gray skies, or feel the trickling tears of the clouds.

The Cactus patient is sad and hypochondriacal; not inclined to speak; weeps quietly but steadily. And for accompanying symptoms there are marked palpitations of the heart, with heavy pressure in the head as if a weight lay on the vertex, and pulsations in the top of the head.

Nux Moschata is a remedy for a melancholy person with hysterical tendencies. The mood is changeable; one moment the patient laughs, and the next cries. Mental activity under Nux Moschata is greatly depressed. The ideas are confused, more so than in Pulsatilla, and there is an inability to continue a train of thought for any length of time. There is loss of memory, and a stupid condition like Anacardium, Opium, and Phosphoric Acid. In speaking or writing, Nux Moschata patients are given to dreamy incoherence of expression.

Digitalis is a remedy that is useful in melancholia with stupor, or in any depressed state when the pulse is slow, and the general circulation throughout the system very stagnant, and when the eyes seem to be brimming with tears.

Gelsemium is called for in melancholia when there is much fever, a general dulness of the mental faculties and a desire to lie in bed and be let alone.

Opium is sometimes used in chronic melancholia when there is vivid imagination, and when the patients are easily frightened; or when there are marked stupidity and hopelessness, with contraction of the pupils.

Veratrum Album is called for in melancholia when physical prostration and mental hopelessness follow an outbreak of maniacal excitement.

Actea Racemosa, Lilium Tigrinum, and Sepia are important remedies in the treatment of melancholic women who are suffering with ovarian or uterine troubles. The mental depression in such cases seems to arise from an abnormal condition of the generative organs. Both Lilium and Sepia are full of apprehensions, and manifest much anxiety for their welfare. In the Sepia case, however, there is likely to be found some serious change in the uterine organs, while the Lilium case presents either functional disturbance, or comparatively superficial organic lesion. Lilium is more applicable to acute cases of melancholia when the uterus or ovaries are involved in moderate inflammation, and when the patient apprehends the presence of a fatal disease which does not exist. The Lilium case quite speedily recovers, much to her own surprise, as well as that of her friends. The Sepia patient is despairing, somewhat suicidal, and averse to work or exercise. This remedy is called for most frequently in cases of long continued uterine disorder, and consequent mental depression.

Actea Racemosa acts in a more general and less specific manner than either Lilium or Sepia. The entire nervous system is affected by the use of Actea, and the condition produced is that of a depressing irritant. The female sexual organs are profoundly impressed by this drug. The menses become erratic and delayed. At the same time the patient feels as if her mind were wrapped in a deep black cloud. She also feels as if she were going cray, and as if death were impending. Intense mental depression, with spasmodic seizures during menstruation, headache in the back of the head, extending over the neck, with rheumatic pains in the muscles of the neck and back, are some of the indications for Actea in melancholia.

We will now consider a few remedies which have been

used successfully for the cure of mania; and, first of all, we will present that medical "Old Guard" composed of the "Big Four" therapeutic veterans—namely, Belladonna, Hyoscyamus, Stramonium, and Veratrum Album.

Probably no remedy in the Materia Medica possesses a wider range of action, or a greater power for relieving distressing symptoms in the brain than Belladonna. Its symptoms are clear and well-defined. Its action is sharp, vigorous, and profound. It is a powerful supplementary ally of Aconite in clearing away the last vestige of cerebral congestion; and beyond this it subdues effectively the subtle process of inflammation. Its symptoms are familar to every student of Materia Medica but it may be well to state, just here, that in a case of insanity where Belladonna is indicated you will find a hot, flushed face (the face is bright red throughout) dilated pupils, throbbing arteries, a fixed and savage look, with now and then sudden spasmodic ebullitions of rage and fury. The Belladonna patient tosses in vague uncertain restlessness. He attempts to bite, strike, tear clothes, strip off clothing, and make outrageous exhibitions of the person, not on account of lecherousness like Cantharis, but because of a disposition to destroy everything that is reachable or tearable. The Belladonna patients are exceedingly fickle, and constantly changing in their mental states. They change suddenly from one mood to another, just as the pain of Belladonna comes suddenly and goes suddenly. They sometimes dance, and sing, and laugh for a short time. But all their moods end in a cyclonic outburst of violence and intolerable rage. Belladonna produces these conditions and symptoms when taken in material doses, and it has relieved, and probably cured, many a case of insanity.

There are two rather opposite conditions existing under the influence of Belladonna. In overprowering doses the

Belladonna patient, after the first period of excitement, becomes dull and heavy, with stertorous breathing, and dark-red besotted countenance, somewhat similar to that of Gelsemium. On the other hand, we find other Belladonna cases exceedingly excitable and nervous, and inclined to move all the time. These are the extreme effects of Belladonna—either a stupid, apoplectic condition on the one hand, and on the other the light, loquacious, active, excited, and restless state of mind. The excitable patient will become quiet under small doses of Belladonna—that is, from the third to the thirtieth potencies, while the stupid patient seems to require a large dose—that is, the first centesimal, or even the first decimal dilution.

Hyoscyamus is a remedy that is called for when there is a lower grade of maniacal excitement than that which calls for Belladonna. The Hyoscyamus patient is very exuberant in his expressions, but less frenzied than the Belladonna case. Hyoscyamus is very talkative, mostly good-natured and jolly. Occasionally he has savage outbursts, and is inclined to be destructive of clothing. The Hyoscyamus patient exposes the person because of lecherous thoughts and obscene tendencies. In this respect Hyoscyamus differs from Belladonna. As I have said, Belladonna tears off clothing for destructiveness; Hyoscyamus tears off clothing for the purpose of exposing the person, and for the purposes of exciting the passions of others. The Hyoscyamus patient is jolly and inclined to talk very much, and for this reason it is a suitable remedy for young, hysterical, nervous, and easily excited women.

The Stramonium patient unites some of the characteristics of Belladonna, Hyoscyamus, and Veratrum Album. The Stramonium case is even more fierce than the Belladonna case. He has laughing fits like Hyoscyamus, or rather like a hyena; he waxes eloquent and pathetic in his despairings of salvation like the prover of Veratrum Album; and he is also greatly troubled with hallucinations. Everything seems to be dark before his eyes. He swears at and makes threats against imaginary foes. He has periods when he is ready and "spoiling for a fight". But for the most part, the Stramonium case is an arrant and crouching coward. He sees animals, of strange varieties and gigantic proportions, leaping at him from the floor or the side-walls, and he is greatly terrified by these apparitions.

Now remember this group of facts: Belladonna is fierce and brave; Hyoscyamus is jolly and companionable; Stramonium is wild and cowardly; Veratrum Album is hopeless and despairing, or wildly plaintive, and beseeching for his salvation, which is apparently lost.

Veratrum Album is a remedy whose sphere of usefulness comprehends both profound prostration of the physical forces, and a most shattered condition of the intellectual faculties. The fame of this drug extends over a period of more than three thousand years. It is related that about the year 1500 before the Christian Era, a certain Melampus, a celebrated physician among the Argives, is said to have cured the daughters of Proteus, King of the Argives, who, in consequence of remaining unmarried, were seized with an "amorous furor" and affected by a "wandering mania". These women had what is now called "old maid's insanity". They were cured chiefly by means of Veratrum Album given in the milk of goats which had been fed upon that plant. We have verified the use of Veratrum Album in "wandering mania" especially when the symptoms of peculiar excitement and tendency to travel are accompanied by great mental distress and physical collapse.

The Veratrum Album patient combines, as primary

effects, the wildest vagaries of the religious enthusiast, the amorous frenzies of the nymphomaniac, and the execrative passions of the infuriated demon, each striving for the ascendency, and causing the unfortunate victim to writhe and struggle with his mental and physical agonies even as the dying Laocoön wrestled with the serpents of Minerva. This anguish is short-lived. The patient soon passes from an exalted and frenzied condition into one of profound melancholia—abject despair of salvation, imbecile taciturnity, and complete prostration of both body and mind. The extremities become cold and blue; the heart's action is weak and irregular; the respiration is hurried, and all the objective symptoms are those of utter collapse. The physical state is like that of a case of cholera. At the same time the mind passes into a stygian gloom from which it slowly, if ever, emerges. With such a picture before us we can scarcely hesitate in the choice of a remedy, and Veratrum Album is the one to be selected. There are, of course, cases which are past the grace of medicine, yet the earnest use of this long-tried drug has frequently repaid us by marked improvement following its administration, and in some cases Veratrum Album has seemed to complete the cure.

We have portrayed a few characteristic symptoms of four drugs for the cure of insanity of the maniacal form. We might add to the list Aconite, with its high fever, its mental anxiety, its restlessness and fear of death. We might also speak of Veratrum Viride which has likewise an exalted temperature, a rapid pulse, great restlessness, fear of being poisoned, and yet withal an indifference to death, which is in sharp contrast with the mental state of Aconite. Veratrum Viride is often indicated in the maniacal attacks to which epileptics and paretics are subject.

Again, we might speak of Nux Vomica, which is a valuable remedy in subacute mania, where the patient is suspicious, and indulges in delusions of persecution and wrong. The Nux Vomica patient is obstinate, incorrigible, cross, ugly, and sometimes studious. Bryonia is also an ugly remedy. The Nux Vomica patient moves about, while the Bryonia patient keeps still because all his symptoms are aggravated by motion.

We might also speak of Lachesis, which is a remedy for those who are extremely sensitive and persistently loquacious, and who indulge in the strange and fantastic idea that they are dead and that preparations for the funeral are going on. The prover of Lachesis feels as if death had overtaken him, because of the profound and depressing effects of that powerful drug. The blood rot of Lachesis is only outrivalled by the blood rot of Baptisia Tinctoria. The victim of the latter thinks that he is all to pieces and scattered about, while Lachesis only thinks that he is dead, and gathered to his fathers.

Rhus Toxicodendron is of service in acute mania when there is a rheumatic history, an excessive restlessness at night, and when the patient is possessed of strong delusions of being poisoned. (Also Hyoscyamus and Veratrum Viride).

Tarantula is a remedy for crafty, cunning maniacs—patients who are full of mischief, and prone to sudden fits of destructiveness, such as knocking down pictures or sweeping bric-a-brac from a mantelpiece, or pounding a piano, or a helpless child.

Sulphur is useful in mania as an intercurrent remedy. Also for "fantastic mania" when the patient decks himself with gaudy colors, and puts on old rags of bright hues, and fancies them the most elegant decorations. Sulphur seldom achieves a cure by itself, but sometimes it seconds with vigor the efforts of other drugs.

When there is great sexual excitement in mania, it may be relieved by the use of Cantharis. The Cantharis patient has frenzied paroxysms of an exalted type like Belladonna. The victim of this remedy bites, and screams, and tears his hair, and howls like a dog. As an invariable accompaniment, there is also great excitement of the sexual organism. In this latter respect, Cantharis resembles Hyoscyamus and Veratrum Album, but these latter drugs commingle the psychical with the physical, the Hyoscyamus patient displaying lively fancies in connection with erotic desires, and the Veratrum Album patient uniting religious sentiment with lustful tendencies; but the Cantharis patient, on the other hand, is strictly and solely the embodiment of lechery for lechery's sake. This is a result of an intense erethism and inflammation of the sexual organs, impelling the victim to seek immediate physical gratification.

Cases of dementia may require Anacardium if the patients are inclined to swear; Apium Virus if the skin is puffy and smooth, and when there is inactivity of the kidneys; Calcarea Carbonica, when patients are fat, flabby and pale; Calcarea Phosphoricum, if there seems to be a tendency to cerebral chilblain; and Phosphoric Acid when the patients are dull and drowsy, with occasional periods of excitement, and profuse discharge of urine. In cases of profound mental depression and mental obfuscation—conditions which suggest both melancholia and dementia—when the nervous system is greatly exhausted, and when there are hysterical tendencies, and when the flow of urine is very profuse, Phosphoric Aci is a leading remedy.

In masturbatic dementia we give Agnus Castus, Causticum, Cantharis, Damiana, Pictric Acid, Phosphorus, Phosphoric Acid, Staphisagria, Nux Vomica, and Opium.

In epileptic dementia we sometimes find Belladonna, Cuprum Aceticum, Laurocerasus, Œnanthe Crocata, and Solanum Carolinense of service in relieving unfortunate symptoms. Œnanthe Crocata has done much good in the relief of epileptic insanity. Solanum Carolinense has been used, but its effects seem to be cumulative, and while the fits may be checked for a season, they return with renewed vigor, and in a dangerous way. Silicea, thirtieth, has been one of the most satisfactory remedies in effecting a wholesome change throughout the general physical system of the patient. As a health-developer in epilepsy, Silicea ranks as one of the first remedies on the list. In medicating epileptics, you should be careful and not overdo the work, and refrain from giving too much medicine. You should regulate the life, the diet, and the exposure to heat and wind. You should encourage the individual to a philosophical and natural state of living. You should provide against the injury of the patient during fits, by covering everything that is hard, and by lining and padding everything which he is likely to strike. All sharp corners should be removed or covered in the room where the epileptic lives. His diet should be plain, wholesome, light, and not stimulating. If you give large doses of medicine and subdue or conceal the fits for a time, you subsequently find that you have simply postponed the evil day. You have worked cumulative damage to your patient, and you have perhaps driven an otherwise quiet and harmless case into the toils of maniacal excitement, or into the deepest and most damnable depths of dementia.

For the relief of general paresis, we may suggest Mercury in its various forms, Nitric Acid, Iodide of Potash; Sulphur and Aurum if syphilis is suspected; and for the relief of the epileptiform seizures, Veratrum Viride, Cimicifuga, Cuprum Metallicum, and Laurocerasus. For the intense restlessness, anxiety, and expansive ideas, together with rapid emaciation of strength and flesh, you may use, according to the symptoms, Aconite, Arsenicum, Belladonna, and Cuprum. Alcohol produces artificial and temporary paresis, and is therefore homeopathic to the genuine article. It may be administered in small doses sometimes with benefit. Good whisky, in one-half ounce doses, may be given once in three or four hours when necessary. These remedies have thus far not proved curative, but have sometimes afforded relief, and have seemed to effect a prolongation of life, and an increased comfort to the sick one.

Hospital Construction

During the past quarter of a century State hospitals for the care and treatment of the insane under homeopathic methods have been established in the commonwealths of New York, Massachusetts, Minnesota, Michigan, California, and Missouri. There should be a public homeopathic hospital for the care of the insane in every state of the Union, because there are believers in that school in every state. Homeopathists pay a considerable proportion of the taxes in each state. If they are denied the privilege of homeopathic treatment when in mental distress, they are suffering not only with disease, but likewise from the condition of taxation without representation. Again, freedom of choice in medical matters is a privilege that is just as sacred to the individual as freedom of choice in any form of religious worship. In order to secure representation wherever there is taxation, and in order to secure absolute freedom of choice in medical matters, you, as physicians, should seek to establish in the state where you live a public hospital where mental invaldis may be treated in accordance with homeopathic principles.

In attaining this desired end, you should consider:

1. A suitable site for the proposed hospital.
2. The economical and durable construction of both large hospital buildings and cottages for the accommodation of the various grades of patients.
3. Ventilation, heating, and lighting.
4. Protection against fire.
5. Furnishings and decorations.
6. Congregate and ward dining-rooms.
7. Kitchen and bakery buildings.
8. Boiler-house, dynamo plant, and laundry.
9. Cold storage building for general supplies.
10. Outbuildings for stock of various kinds.

Site.—In selecting the site for a hospital you should seek the moderate hilltops or sunny slopes of protecting mountains, although you should at the same time consider the difficulty of getting coal, water, and provisions to their destination without unnecessary expense. You should, if possible, locate the buildings in such a place that you may have railroad communication direct to the institution; thus the hospital will be subjected to no heavy expense for long cartage of coal, or other materials. A little oversight on this point would lead, perhaps, to a subsequent expenditure of thousands of dollars per year, and without any real necessity for it.

Sites suitable for good sanitation must be attained, but to these may properly be added the inspirations of grand and stirring scenery of either the summits or the surf. Patients who are convalescing from insanity are stimulated and helped to recovery by the beauty or grandeur of the environments which nature throws about them. It is said that sea air has a soporific influence upon patients suffering with mania, while the air and scenery of the mountains are most inspiring and beneficial to the victims of melancholia.

The soil of the site selected should be dry and porous, or if it is a stiff clay, it should at least be amenable to the influence of good drainage and cultivation.

Building.—The buildings designed for the care of the insane should be located due north and south, or a little east of south, in order to secure throughout the year as much sunshine as possible upon the east, south, and west sides of the buildings.

After many experiments, it has been determined that hospital buildings for the insane should be not more than two stories in height. The buildings should be of moderate size, each accommodating from twenty to one hundred and fifty patients. Buildings of moderate size can be furnished with light and fresh air more readily than large buildings, and patients can be more easily classified in small buildings than in large ones.

A public institution designed for the accommodation of twelve hundred or fifteen hundred patients may properly consist of a series of buildings of moderate size, and these, for convenience of access, and for the ready distribution of food, may be connected with each other by suitable corridors. If the site is large enough, it is well to erect the buildings on the borders of a large rectangle or parallelogram. Within the general enclosure of buildings and corridors designed for patients may be situated a boiler house, a dynamo plant, a laundry, a kitchen and bakery, an entertainment hall, and a library. In this country, where changes in the weather are frequent and at times very pronounced, it is better to have the institution so constructed that the patients may go from all the wards to the library and the entertainment hall and chapel without being obliged to suffer any exposure in the open air. By means of suitable corridors from one building to another, the officers and employees are also protected in the discharge of duty from unfavourable weather.

The buildings should be constructed of brick with hollow walls, and they should be sufficiently strong for all practical purposes. The floors should be built of steel girders and brick arches, overlaid with tile in the water-sections, and panelled oak or body maple in the wards. The ceilings should be of steel fashioned into bright and attractive patterns, or the brick arches may be plastered and painted. The side walls should be of adamant cement, and every corner should be made a quarter-round.

Each building should have a basement not less than nine feet in height, and it should come well out of the ground, in order that it may at all times be supplied with fresh air, and as much sunshine as possible. The floor of the basement should be of cement or stone. The basement floor should be laid in a sloping fashion toward the drain, so that the basement may be cleansed by hosing water over the floors and into the drain pipes.

The hospital building should be divided into large roms, each containing thirty to seventy-five or more beds. A few single rooms should be provided in each hospital building. The hospital or reception wards should be spacious and airy, with high ceilings and numerous windows. Every hospital ward should be provided with a solarium, or sunroom, where the patients may secure the beneficial effects of sunlight and fresh air at all times, and under the most favourable circumstances. The open wards may contain most of the patients, while the single rooms can be used for the disturbed or the very sensitive. Each ward should have easy access to a tower containing baths, lavatories, water-closets, urinals, and slop sinks.

If it seems necessary to isolate some very disturbed cases, they may be placed in one-story hospital buildings detached from the main structures. These buildings should be thoroughly lighted and, if necessary, skylights, as well as side-lights, may be used. But there are very few disturbed cases nowadays who do not become quiet more quickly if associated with others than if kept in absolute seclusion. The seclusion of the noisy and the violent should be only a temporary matter. We think that at least sixty-five per cent of the acute insane may be properly treated in large hospital wards in association with each other, and where trained nurses may have their eyes upon all the patients all the time, both day and night. By such means the patients get constant nursing, and the method is economical, as a nurse can take better care of half a dozen patients if they are in one room, than he can of three patients if they are isolated in single rooms. It is thought by some that when a large number of patients are placed in one ward they will disturb and annoy each other. This supposition is not founded upon fact, because each patient is so absorbed in his own throughts that he pays but little heed to the thoughts and expressions of others. Hence the insane do as well when they are in hospital wards as when they are confined in small single rooms; in fact, it seems to me that the majority do better under the conditions of association. Occasionally there is a patient who does not harmonize with his fellows, or even tolerate them, and in such a case a small private room should be afforded. Each person should be considered from an individual standpoint, and he should be favored with such surroundings as are most likely to insure his speedy recovery. When patients begin to convalesce, they sometimes desire to seek the seclusion which is afforded by a single room. When they have secured all the benefits of treatment in a general hospital ward, then they should be granted the privilege of a room by themselves, or a room in which two or three patients can be happily associated.

Patients who have partially recovered in reception wards may be transferred to other suitable wards, or to cottages which are adapted to the care of such cases. In wards and cottages for convalescent and recovering patients, it is often feasible to practice what is called the "open-door system". The doors are unlocked during the daytime, and the patients go out and come in at their pleasure, after their tendencies have been observed, and their trustworthiness ascertained as fully as possible by the attending physician. No patient should be permitted to have an unrestricted parole until his mental condition is such that he can appreciate the benefit and feel the responsibility of such freedom.

If the hospital buildings are two stories in height, then the floors should be thoroughly deafened, in order to prevent the patients on the second floor from disturbing those on the first, by shouting or dancing above them.

Ventilation, Heating, and Lighting.—There are several methods of enforcing ventilation in a hospital ward, but the sum and substance of them all is embodied in the one word "draught". The foul air must be made to move out, and the fresh air must be made to come in, and these exchanges of impure for pure air all depend upon the laws of motion.

The vital questions to be decided are:

1. How swift shall be the current of moving air; and,
2. How frequently shall the air in a hospital be entirely changed?

A rapid draught may cause discomfort, or even dangers to the patients. Rapid draughts of cold air induce attacks of influenza, bronchitis, and pneumonia. If the volume of air moves too slowly through a hospital ward, then there is danger that some of the impurities may remain, and thus produce disease. It is claimed that the best and safest rate of motion of air in a ward is about two miles per hour. Much, however, depends upon the condition of the air itself—its temperature, and its humidity. In summer ventilation may be secured through windows and doors. The best method of window ventilation is to raise the lower sash about six or eight inches, and let down the upper sash about the same distance. Much of the impure air is lighter than common air; hence these impurities escape if the upper sash is lowered. The currents of fresh air coming in through the lower opening facilitate the transmission of foul air to the upper regions. Sometimes the air becomes laden with carbonic acid gas, and this being heavier than common air settles to the floor. In removing this heavy foul air, the advantages of doors and French windows are plainly apparent. With a door on one side of the room and a French window on the other, the foul air that is heavier than common air is easily swept away. The best ventilation by means of windows and doors would be secured if each room or ward were supplied with long doors on one side, and French windows, on the other. These, when opened wide, favor the free passage of air, and if there are enough of these windows the atmosphere in a ward soon becomes like the atmosphere out-of-doors—entirely pure, and free from odors.

It should be the aim of all who are in charge of hospitals for the sick to keep the air of the wards as pure and fresh as that which is uncovered by any roof, and which has been made fresh and invigorating by the cleansing blows of the pelting storm, and the actinic rays of the noonday sun.

MEDICAL TREATMENT

In winter the proper ventilation of wards and hospitals is a more difficult task to accomplish than during the summer. During the cold season ventilation must be associated with the heating apparatus. Fresh air should be sent into the wards by passing it over hot steam coils or pipes filled with hot water. Foul air must be taken away through conduits extending to the attic, and these should be connected with a large cylinder supplied with steam pipes, to rarify the air and produce a draught; and above the cylinder there should be constructed suitable ventilators for the exit of the impure and exhausted air of the wards. By means of a suitable steam-heating apparatus, fresh air may be driven into the wards constantly, and foul air may be drawn out of the wards by the means already referred to. The impure air is rarified by heat, and drawn up through pipes or hollow tubing, until it reaches the peak of the attic, and thence it passes into the open air through suitable ventilators.

While the air in a hospital ward can be properly heated and systematically distributed, and while the impurities, as a rule, may be drawn up and forced out at the top of the building, yet we believe that the French window and the open-door system of changing absolutely and completely all the air in the ward should be resorted to from time to time. By the ordinary process of heating and ventilation, the air is, for the most part, kept in a fairly pure state, but some of the fresh air is constantly coming in contact with the impure air which has not yet wholly departed, and consequently there remain, even in a well-ventilated ward, some of its native and inherent impurities. These can be removed only by an absolute, speedy and complete change, by opening all the sides of the house, so to speak, at suitable intervals—that is, by opening the French windows and the doors.

The heating of a hospital building may be carried on by the indirect method, or by the direct-indirect, or by the direct method. By the indirect method the steam coils are all kept in the basement, and thus space is economized in the ward. The indirect method is best for violent, or disturbed, or epileptic patients, as such patients are less liable to be injured by the indirect method of heating than by the direct. When the radiators are in the wards the epileptic patients almost inevitably fall upon them when having fits; and now and then a violent patient will attack a radiator when it is hot as if it were an enemy, and in that way he gets burned.

The direct-indirect method of heating is a combination of direct heating, and ventilation from out of doors. The same objections apply to it as to the direct method.

The indirect method is probably the best, except that it may have to be supplemented in cold corners of the building by carrying the steam direct to these exposed points. The steam-heating of hospital buildings has been carried to a very satisfactory pitch of perfection, and this method of heating will probably continue until superseded by electricity.

Some prefer the hot water method of heating, but this system requires an excessive amount of large pipes, and these occupy much space, and that would be a serious objection if it were desirable to use the direct method of heating. In case a pipe breaks in a system where hot water is used for heating, the flooding of the rooms and wards might be an additional objection.

Every hospital should be abundantly supplied with sunlight during the day, and to this end large windows and plenty of them are needed. During the evening the wards should be favored with an ample number of electric lights. These lights should be covered with suitable shades, to protect the eyes of the patients. Except during the sleeping hours, all gloom should be dispelled as far as possible by the introduction of light in almost unlimited quantities. Darkness favours a continuance of gloomy thoughts, while light tends to restore hope and happiness to the human soul.

Protection Against Fire—Every hospital should be scrupulously protected against the ravages of fire. Such protection is a prime necessity. In each large public hospital there should be a well organized fire brigade. The members of this brigade should consist of those who work in the engineer's department, and of the attendants and nurses who work upon the wards. They should be regularly drilled at frequent intervals in the handling of apparatus to be used for the putting out of fires.

There should be in each hospital a system of electric fire alarms, so constructed as to reveal, at the outset, the exact location of the fire. There should be an abundant water supply for fire purposes, and it should be distributed by means of pipes through every ward, and by means of hydrants on every side of each building exteriorly. Each institution should have a hose house, with an abundance of hose rolled upon carriages. Everything that is needful for the speedy attachment of the hose to the hydrants, in case of conflagration, should be furnished, and kept in the most convenient place. A portable chemical fire engine is also a desirable addition to the fire apparatus.

In addition to the foregoing, each ward of each building should be supplied with portable fire extinguishers of approved pattern and tested capability. Hand grenades, fire pails, water in barrels and tubs should also be provided, and within easy reach of the employees, especially at night.

Above and beyond all the measures heretofore suggested, we believe that a system of automatic fire sprinklers should be installed in every room, and every ward, and every basement, and every attic of every building devoted to the care of the insane. The greatest horror that can befall an institution where the helpless sick is housed is the calamity of fire. It is almost impossible to put out a fire when once fairly started. Each ventilating shaft, or clothes chute, or elavator passageway, becomes, in the hour of fire, a chimney through which the flames are forced with a draught that equals the most elaborate and scientific boiler-house smokestack. Hence, when a fire is once started, it is, as we have remarked, almost impossible to check it. Therefore, it becomes our duty to prevent fires rather than to indulge in the almost useless task of trying to put them out after they are once started. Every new building designed for the care of the insane should be protected by a method known as the "automatic fire extinguishing system". This system consists of a series of pipes which pass to every ward and room in each building. At proper intervals these automatic sprinklers are placed, and when any one of them is brought to a heat of 160°F., a cap, which is held in place by soft solder, is released, and a most vigorous diffusion of spray follows. This spray strikes the ceiling, the side-walls, and the floors, and is generally successful in extinguishing all incipient fires. This system does not rely upon the tardy discoveries of a sleepy night-watch, but it works without direction or command, vigorously and effectively whenever and wherever the first flames of a kindling conflagration bring the heat of a room or hall to 160°F. The automatic fire sprinkler is probably the best and safest means for the prevention of large fires, by putting out the small ones while they are yet in an incipient stage of development.

There should also be provision made in every hospital for the speedy and safe escape of inmates from the buildings in case a fire should occur. If future structures designed for the insane shall be only two stories in height, then the danger from fire will be lessened. But in any event, it is wise to prepare beforehand for every possible disaster. We have examined into the merits of several varieties of fire escapes, ranging from the simple iron ladder to an elaborate and wire-protected iron stairway. Down the latter when wide enough, sick patients may be carried on cots, if they are unable to walk. But a fire escape composed of iron "treads and risers" is liable, in time of fire, to be filled with smoke and flame, in which case it is almost impossible to utilize it in those conditions.

Probably the best fire escape is a cylinder of steel about six feet in diameter. The outer shell is composed of steel plates tightly riveted together. Within is a spiral chute. This chute is fastened to and supported by the external cylinder. In the center is an iron pipe which may be used as a conduit for water. The chute is fastened centrally to this pipe. The cylinder is attached to the building in such a way as to be easily accessible from each floor. Down this steel spiral structure patients may slide very rapidly without danger to themselves or others. It is said that one hundred persons may escape from a burning building in one minute through a chute of this kind. People enter the cylinder by passing through two iron doors, one closing behind the person before the second is opened. This keeps back the smoke and flame to a very large extent. If the fire reaches and heats the cylinder at any point, it may be cooled from without by the application of a stream of water.

Furnishings and Decorations.—The furniture for the use of the insane should be strong but comfortable, and of a pattern that will appear neat, that can be readily cleaned, and that will not harbor vermin. The bedstead should be of iron with woven wire spring; and the mattress should be either of the best of hair, or the best of cotton felt. The cotton felt mattress of proper quality is pliable and soft, and does not get lumpy or mat like a hair mattress. For these reasons the felt mattress seems to me to be the most appropriate for bed patients. Patients who are constantly in bed, upon hair mattresses are apt to have their skins irritated by the occasional protrusion through the mattress of a sharp end of a stiff and half-curled hair. This does not occur when the best of elastic cotton felt is used.

Each hospital should be furnished, aside from a bed and table for each patient, with large, easy rocking chairs, and invalid chairs. We do not, however, advocate the use of upholstered furniture, except in the sitting-rooms of wards for the accommodation of convalescent patients; for the reason that it is quite easily soiled, and the expense of keeping it in good condition is therefore considerable.

The furnishings and decorations of each room should constitute an harmonious individuality by itself, and yet all the rooms should be made to harmonize with the ward. We think that the walls should be painted in light colors, because they are more soothing than dark colors. Pictures should be placed upon the walls, and curtains at the windows of both sitting-rooms and bed-rooms. A mistaken notion prevails that insane patients often destroy such furnishings, but experience has tended to prove the contrary. Only a very small percentage of such patients destroy beautiful furniture or furnishings. Rugs are preferable to carpets, as they are more easily kept clean. Furnishings of a bright and inspiring character not only tend to the beautifying of a ward, but they may be classed as positive curative agents. The lively interest which the patients take in any new furniture that is placed upon a ward is sometimes really remarkable.

Congregate or Ward Dining-rooms.—Much has been written during the past twenty years about associate or congregate dining-rooms. In institutions having two thousand or three thousand patients, the interests of economy are conserved by erecting large dining-rooms convenient to the wards, and also adjacent to the kitchen building. Thus the food may be served hot and promptly, with the smallest practical number of attendants. These large dining-rooms are very convenient and satisfactory for the chronic insane who are able to be up and dressed, and who can easily walk from the ward to the dining-room; but for patients suffering with acute insanity, who are obliged to remain in the hospital wards, and much of the time in bed, the congregate dining-room is, it seems to me, unavailable. Attached to every hospital ward should be a convenient pantry and a small dining-room, where the food may be quickly served when sent from the kitchen. In every hospital for mental invalids there is quite a considerable number of patients who are sensitive as to their surroundings. These should be placed in wards of moderate size, and there should be a small dining-room attached to each one of these wards. These patients may then be classified in such a manner as to best conserve their general welfare, and make them as happy as possible. A dozen congenial patients may sit down at a table in a small room and enjoy their meals, while if they were forced to eat in a large congregate dining-room, where the table manners of some are highly objectionable, they would be unable to take food in sufficient and satisfying quantities. I believe that every institution should be provided with large dining-rooms and small dining-rooms, arranged in such a manner as to insure the best interests and the greatest possible comfort of all concerned.

The objection to small dining-rooms is that they require more help in the aggregate than the large dining-rooms. But these small dining-rooms can be looked after in such a manner as to be reasonably economical in their management. The attendants in small dining-rooms as soon as their work is finished (and that is quickly done by the help of patients) may then engage in the task of exercising patients out-of-doors, and in performing such other duties as may properly be assigned to them.

Kitchen and Bakery Building.—The kitchen and bakery building should be separate from all other buildings, aside from store rooms and cold storage. There should be a narrow corridor connecting this building with the basements of the other hospital structures, and through which the food car may pass. The kitchen and bakery building should be large, light and roomy, and as nearly as possible fireproof. The floors should be of Porland cement, put down upon a solid and unchanging foundation. The building should be so arranged as to receive all raw material at one side of the structure, and the food, after it has been prepared, should be sent out to the wards from the other side of the building. The scullery should be so situated that all soiled utensils coming back from the wards may be washed before they get to the kitchen or bakery again. The kitchen furniture should be capacious enough for all possible needs of the hospital; and the boilers and ranges should be set up in such a manner as to be convenient of access to those who must prepare the food. Lack of room in the cooking establishment of an institution, or inconvenience of arrangement, will tend to produce unnecessary strain upon the workers, and this will finally result in carelessness in one of the most important of all hospital tasks—namely, the proper preparation of food.

Boiler-house, Dynamo Plant, and Laundry.—The various buildings for heating, lighting, and laundry work should be commodious and convenient. The tendency at the outset is almost always toward a too rigid economy, and a miserly stringency of space. It is unwise to put up small buildings for an institution which may in time, by the addition of various wings and wards, come to accommodate two thousand or more patients. These necessary adjuncts to hospital wards should be made fireproof and they should be situated in the rear of the main building, and as nearly as possible in the center of the inner court—that is, if the hospital wards are grouped about a large rectangle. If the linear plan of construction is pursued, then these various buildings should be in the rear of the main or administrative building. For purposes of safety, and to avoid annoying the sick, the boiler-house, dynamo plant and laundry should be located at least three hundred or four hundred feet from the wards.

Cold Storage Building.—A cold storage building is now considered an essential necessity for the preservation of meat, milk, butter, eggs, vegetables, fruit, and other perishable articles. With a cold storage the authorities of an institution may take advantage of low market rates at certain seasons of the year, and lay in a large supply as cheaply as practicable. This building should be convenient of access to the kitchen and bakery, and large enough to hold a three months' supply of food at the least.

Outbuildings for Stock of Various Kinds.—It seems to

be the policy of the various states to have a farm in connection with each State hospital, hence there is a necessity for barns, and stables, and piggeries, and other buildings for the accommodation of the various kinds of stock. The task of caring for horses, cows, pigs, chickens and ducks may be carried on successfully by the aid of convalescent and intelligent patients. These outbuildings should be located so far away from the hospital that they cannot become sources of annoyance to the patients.

The task of upbuilding a public institution for the insane is a noble and a glorious one. It is an undertaking worthy of the attention, the careful contemplation, and the best energies of any thoughtful man. The upbuilding of an establishment, whose outlines we have endeavored very briefly to sketch, is an enterprise so lofty in purpose, and so beneficent in result as to afford serene satisfaction to all who may engage in the work.

In the heart of London, England, there stands a magnificent structure known as St. Paul's Cathedral. The architect of this gigantic and stately edifice was Sir Christopher Wren. When his great work was completed, he inscribed upon the rim of the grand dome in the center of the cathedral this word, "*Circumspice*", which means in plain English, "Look around".

When the modern hospital is completed upon the plans outlined in this lecture, then all the people may be invited to "look around", and behold with pleasure the results attained when benevolence and philanthropy, enlightened intelligence and enthusiastic energy, unite their forces for the purpose of effecting that which is best in the care and comfort and cure of mental invalids.

COMPENDIUM

We present herewith, alphabetically, a list of remedies for mental disorders, with characteristic mental and allied symptoms.

ACONITE

General Action.—Aconite affects primarily the cerebro-spinal and sympathetic ganglionic systems. It stimulates the inhibitory centers of the pneumogastric, and by hyper-stimulation the pneumogastric nerve becomes exhausted, as is shown by the heart's action becoming quickened and more irregular, until finally paralysis of the heart may occur. Aconite, when given in large doses, produces inevitable cardiac depression and a tendency to death. In less poisonous doses, this drug produces acute inflammatory action throughout the system. The precise manner in which the inflammatory process is induced by Aconite has not been satisfactorily explained, but it has been suggested that by causing paralysis of the vasomotor nerves, the arterioles dilate, doubling their capacity, and thus patients are bled, so to speak, in their own vessels. Wherever there is an excessive supply of blood, there is a tendency to inflammatory metamorphosis.

Brain and Spinal Cord.—Congestion of the brain, with oversensitiveness to light; heat and redness of the face, or pale face; carotids pulsate strongly; pulse full and strong (also Belladonna, Gelsemium, Veratrum Viride); headache as if the brain were moved or raised; burning in the forehead as if in boiling water; vertigo; conjunctivitis; pupils contracted or dilated; formication over the spine; numbness of spine; spasms from inflammation of spine; numbness and tingling of limbs; paralysis of limbs; jerking of arm and leg; nausea and vomiting of cerebral origin; the least noise, especially of music, aggravates the brain symptoms.

Mind.—Great fear of approaching death; inconsolable anguish; dread of men; fear of ghosts; fears the loss of reason; mental prostration, with weakness of memory; cannot remember dates; changing mood, from dry anguish to exuberant tears; the mind suffers from the effects of anger or fright.

Sleep.—Sleeplessness, with anxiety and mental restlessness.

Accompaniments.—Full hard pulse and flushed face; hypertrophy of the heart; pain in the cardiac region; and pain and tingling in the left arm.

Special Sphere of Action.—Aconite is indicated for the restless mental anxiety in the victims of intense shock. The state calling for Aconite is one of anguish, anxiety, and nervous excitement. It has a marked influence upon the cerebral circulation, and is useful for cases in which formerly venesection was prescribed. In threatened apoplexy and apoplectiform seizures, when there are congestion of the brain, vertigo, flushed face and thick speech, and when there are intense anxiety and restlessness, Aconite will often dispel or relieve these morbid symptoms, and sometimes apparently avert an attack. Experience in repeated cases has verified its usefulness under these conditions. In mania and melancholia, with intense restlessness, due to mental anxiety and nervous excitement, with great fear of death, whether the condition is accompanied by fever or not, particularly in acute cases with marked sthenic symptoms, beginning with great violence, and when symptoms are worse at evening, a few doses of Aconite, given at short intervals during the early part of the night, will often procure for the patient a natural and restful sleep.

Aconite is of great service in the convulsions of paresis; also in those rapidly occurring convulsions of epilepsy which constitute the *status epilepticus*. Here Aconite seems to afford the relief which is said to follow the removal of the cerebro-spinal fluid by lumbar puncture.

Almost daily, by the use of this drug, we are able to check beginning inflammatory conditions caused by exposure to unusually cold draughts, and the early use of this drug in such cases is doubtless one reason why, at this hospital, there has been so little pneumonia in the past twenty-five years.

AGARICUS MUSCARIUS

General Action.—This fungus is classed by toxicologists as a narcotic, acrid poison (Christison). It acts upon the blood, rendering it fluid, so that it runs easily from the bodies of those killed by it; it produces gangrene in the stomach and intestines.

Brain and Spinal Cord.—Agaricus produces congestion of the brain, with stupidity; heaviness of the head as if intoxicated; the spine is sensitive to touch; there are severe burning pains in the spine, with jerkings or tremblings of the facial and cervical muscles.

Mind.—Confusion of mind; unable to find the right word when speaking (compare Alumina, Calcarea Carbonica, Chamomilla, and Lycopodium); disinclined to answer questions; sings and talks, but will not answer when spoken to; indisposed to perform any labor, especially mental; ill-humored and irritable; merry and singing in ecstasies; and again prostrated by general malaise; people who are solicitous and anxious about ordinary affairs become, under the effects of Agaricus, moody and indifferent to their surroundings.

Sleep.—Irresistible drowsiness in the daytime; on falling asleep the muscles of the body twitch suddenly, and the patient awakens.

Accompaniments.—Severe pains in the stomach; grass-green diarrhoeic stools; cutting pains in the abdomen, and sometimes dysenteric discharges.

Special Sphere of Action.—Paretic conditions after sexual and other debauches; mental obtuseness, with ill-humor; trembling and twitching of groups of muscles; coma following febrile or mental excitement; general paresis, mania and primary dementia.

ALUMINA

General Action.—The most characteristic effects of this substance are evidenced in motor weakness and sensory disturbance of the lower extremities, and in extreme dryness and irritation of the mucous membranes. The secretions are thick, scanty, and acrid.

Brain and Spinal Cord.—Stitching burning pain in the head, with vertigo, worse in the morning, but relieved by food. Burning pain in the spine, as though pierced by a hot iron; numbness of the legs, as though walking on cushions. Arms and legs heavy, as though paralyzed; legs weak and easily tired; cannot walk without the aid of vision.

Mind.—Low-spirited and hypochondriacal; little obstacles seem insurmountable; is peevish, whining and always ready to give up. Thoughts of suicide are suggested by the sight of possible means of its accomplishment, but are repugnant, and contribute to the patient's suffering. Time seems long; joy in work is gone; the consciousness of personality is obscured; memory fails; and complete loss of reason is dreaded. These symptoms grow better as the day advances.

Sleep.—Lassitude during the day, with an inclination to lie down. At night is restless, and disturbed by anxious dreams; awakens with palpitation of the heart.

Accompaniments.—Dyspepsia, with capricious appetite; rejects nourishing food, and wants unusual and indigestible articles. Constipation, dry stools passed by great straining. Atrophic catarrhs of the upper respiratory passages, with scant, thick, tough, yellow mucus; ropy tenacious leucorrhea; conjunctivitis, the lids are cracked and stiff.

Special Sphere of Action.—Alumina is most useful in persons of advanced years, spare and wrinkled, and illy nourished. It is indicated in the milder types of melancholia, accompanied by considerable confusion of mind, and a tendency to chronicity. It has an extensive use in the spinal degenerations and paralysis of the lower limbs, particularly in locomotor ataxia.

ANACARDIUM

General Action.—Anacardium depresses the intellectual centers and the organs of special sense, with sensation of general weakness and faintness.

Brain and Spinal Cord.—Severe, tearing, nervous headache, or as though a plug were forced into the brain, usually on the left side.

Mind.—Great weakness or total loss of memory. Recollection of single names presents the greatest difficulty. Irritable and passionate; irresistible desire to curse and swear. It sometimes seems to the distracted patient as though he had two separate wills swaying him in opposite directions; cannot apply the mind; hallucinations; seems to hear the voices of absent relatives, or to smell filth ever before the nose, especially when smelling the clothes or body.

Sleep.—Great sleepiness during the day; mostly in the forenoon.

Accompaniments.—Pain as if a plug were forced into various parts of the body, especially in the rectum, with constipation. Frequently hungry; feels better while eating, but aggravated afterward.

Special Sphere of Action.—Anacardium relieves nervous headache, the result of overexertion, and the weakness of memory and inability to think which result from exhausting physical disease, or which immediately follow the more violent symptoms of the acute psychoses; and it is sometimes used, though with much less success, because of the organic nature of the disease, in the various forms of terminal dementia.

ANTIMONIUM CRUDUM

General Action.—The antimonial salts attack the mucous membranes, especially the lining of the gastro-intestinal canal, producing vomiting, and in poisonous doses purging, with profound depression of the vital powers.

Brain and Spinal Cord.—Heaviness in the head, with vertigo. Headache increased by going up stairs (also Calcarea Carbonica).

Mind.—Cross and peevish; if only looked at is angry, sulky, and wants no communication with any one; sentimental; has amorous longings, not for any living creature, but for some unseen seraph boded forth by an ecstatic imagination.

Sleep.—Sleepiness during the forenoon; sleeps heavily, but is unrefreshed.

Accompaniments.—Thickening and irregular growth of the skin and nails. The tongue is covered with a uniform white coating. Watery diarrhea, especially in hot weather, containing little lumps of fecal matter, with vomiting of food, and anorexia.

Special Sphere of Action.—It is suited to the mental condition of some young persons passing through the critical pubescent period, whose growing interest in the opposite sex tends to center unhealthfully in some bright Prince Charming, or in some idealized, and perhaps entirely self-created maiden. Moderate, regular occupation; plenty of exercise in the open air; frequent association with other boys and girls of a similar age under simple natural conditions, and attention to the character of the literature read, are cardinal accessories in the management of such a case.

ANTIMONIUM TARTARICUM

General Action.—Similar to Antimonium Crudum, with more nausea and retching, and greater circulatory depression. The heart's action is feeble; the pulse soft and tremulous.

Brain and Spinal Cord.—Its characteristic effects on the lungs, heart, liver, and stomach are brought about by its action upon the origin of the pneumogastric nerve. There is headache as if a band were compressing the forehead. (Mercurius, Nitric Acid, and Sulphur have the sensation of a hoop bound tightly around the head.)

Mind.—Restless and apprehensive; does not want to be left alone, yet cannot bear to be touched.

Sleep.—Yawning; irresistible desire to sleep; awakened often by abdominal disturbance.

Accompaniments.—Inflammation of the smaller bronchi, much rattling of mucus in the chest; numerous fine bubbling râles; oppression of breathing; blueness of the surface and cardiac failure; green watery diarrhea (Veratrum Album). A pustular eruption on the skin.

Special Sphere of Action.—Antimonium Tartaricum is a remedy little called for in treating the strictly mental manifestations of the insane, but of frequent us in combating their physical ills. In capillary bronchitis it should be given early, not, as often the case, administered only after the rattling of death is heard in the throat, and no remedy can succeed. It is also of use in the gastric and intestinal disorders which may follow when patients with impaired judgment overload the stomach, as they will so frequently do if not watchfully guarded by an intelligent and observing nurse.

APIS MELLIFICA

General Action.—It defibrinates the blood, and causes inflammation of a low grade, in which the tissues rapidly break down and become gangrenous; it also causes serous effusions. These blood changes produce mental stupidity, and often coma.

Brain and Spinal Cord.—Hydrocephalus, with piercing shrieks; vertigo, worse lying down (also Conium); coma, with constant jerkings of the limbs; stinging pains in the back.

Mind.—Stupidity, absent-mindedness, awkwardness; lets things drop from the hands (also Hellebore); loss of memory; moody; irritable; jealous (also Hyoscyamus); mania from sexual excitement in women; fear of death, with sensations that they are going to die.

Sleep.—Great inclination to sleep, but cannot do so because of mental restlessness (Aconite and Coffea); cramping and starting in sleep; unpleasant dreams; dreams of flying and journeying.

Accompaniments.—Erysipelatous condition of the face; pain, and tenderness, and dropsy of the ovaries, especially the right; scanty micturition, and sometimes a general dropsical condition.

Special Sphere of Action.—Mental stupidity, with occasional periods of restlessness and screaming; jealousy in women who suffer with sharp pains in the ovaries, especially in the right.

ARGENTUM NITRICUM

General Action.—It leads to destruction of the coloring matter of the red corpuscles; profound anemia and malnutrition, followed by destructive inflammations of the bones and periosteum; cerebro-spinal disturbances, and fatty degeneration of the muscles and glandular organs.

Brain and Spinal Cord.—Tetanic convulsions, paralysis, coma, and death from asphyxia follow the administration of large doses. Headache deep in the brain, or as if the cranial bones were expanding (also Glonoin). Better with tight band around the head (also Silicea). Spinal pains and weakness; limbs are weak and imperfectly coordinated, with vertigo, and trembling nervous weakness.

Mind.—Irresolute and melancholic; hesitates to undertake anything from fear of failure (also Arnica). Feels as if under a mental cloud (compare Cimicifuga); and has no interest in ordinary employments. The memory is poor.

Sleep.—Restless; anxious, frightful dreams which seem true on awakening.

Accompaniments.—Pain in the pit of the stomach, which radiates in all directions; belching of large quantities of wind; facial neuralgia, with a sour taste in the mouth; asthma; spasms of the respiratory muscles; throat sore, dark red, and swollen; purulent ophthalmia.

Special Sphere of Action.—It is useful in cases of hypochondriasis and mental failure, accompanied by flatulent or nervous dyspepsia, or caused by overindulgence in the use of alcohol, and excesses in venery. It is indicated and successfully used in locomotor ataxia, and to a less extent in other forms of sclerosis of the brain and spinal cord. Epileptic convulsions followed by tremor have also been cured by its administration.

ARNICA

General Action.—It slows up the action of the heart, and raises the arterial pressure. There is capillary stasis, and a tendency to hemorrhages in the brain.

Brain and Spinal Cord.—Left-sided paralysis from concussion; tired, weary feeling in the head, worse on lying down; sensation that everything feels hard.

Mind.—The Arnica patient has fits of anguish or hopeless indifference; forgets what he is reading, or the word he is about to use (Anacardium, Lilium Tigrinum, Lycopodium); fears being struck by persons coming near him; easily frightened; unexpected troubles make him start; answers questions very slowly, sometimes falling asleep while answering.

Accompaniments.—Bladder affections of traumatic origin; tenesmus, with spasms of the neck of the bladder; general prostration from blows upon any part of the body.

Special Sphere of Action.—Arnica is useful in cases resulting from traumatism, particularly when mental disturbance is traceable to injury about the head, even though the injury occurred several years previously. Schrœder Van der Kolk claims that Arnica is invaluable in certain cases of mania when the first excitement has passed, and there remain a heat in the head, and a tendency to imbecility. Arnica is also of use after apoplectiform seizures and paralytic symptoms which remain after apoplexy. The patient manifests weakness of memory, and confusion of mind; is absent-minded, complains of a bruised, sore feeling, especially after concussion. This sensation of soreness, as though from a bruise, is characteristic of Arnica.

ARSENICUM

General Action.—Arsenicum acts upon the ganglionic nervous system; it acts upon the mucous and serous membranes, producing in the former especially, inflammation of a low grade. There is a marked tendency, under Arsenicum, of the tissues to become gangrenous; also there are effusions into those cavities which are lined by serous membranes.

Brain and Spinal Cord.—The nervous system is apparently affected, reflexly, by the disturbance of the digestive apparatus; there is frontal headache, and the pains are of a burning character; there are vertigo and *tinnitus aurium*; sensitiveness and burning in spine.

Mind.—Melancholia; and tearful and depressed mood; intense anxiety, with great restlessness; fears to be left alone lest he should do himself bodily harm; great fear, with cold sweats; cannot find rest anywhere; wants to move from bed to bed; is intensely suicidal and is inclined to mutilate the body; the patient has hallucinations of smell; smells pitch and sulphur, and anticipates consignments to Sheol.

Sleep.—Sleeplessness, with restlessness and anxiety; frequent starting in sleep; awakened by pain, especially after midnight; after sleep feels as if he had not slept enough; dreams full of care, sorrow and fear, about thunderstorms, fire, black water, and death.

Accompaniments.—Asthmatic conditions; difficulty in respiration; thirst for small quantities of water at frequent intervals; weakness and palpitation of the heart; emaciation of the body, followed by dropsical tendencies; scanty urine, and burning during micturition.

Special Sphere of Action.—Arsenicum finds a variety of application among the insane in affections characterized by periodicity, great weakness and prostration, symptoms of a malign nature, restlessness and anguish, burning sensations, unquenchable thirst for small quantities of water, and, very often, pains which are worse at rest, and increased by cold. It is useful when the patient is delirious, depressed, restless, has fear of death, fear of being alone, and has strong suicidal tendencies. There is often noticed a tendency among the insane to mutilation of the body; picking the skin until it is sore, and chewing the finger nails. Here Arsenicum relieves. This drug causes intense prostration; hence it is useful in those cases of acute delirious mania and exhaustive insanity which are accompanied by typhoid symptoms and by rapid emaciation. We note especially its good effects upon the victims of resistive and restless melancholia, of active and ever-strring mania, and of rapidly failing paresis. Dr. Hughes states that Arsenicum is one of the few remedies which causes genuine neuralgia, and far excels all other remedies in the treatment of idiopathic disorder. There is intense sensitiveness of the scalp under Arsenicum. This drug is said to produce epilepsy, with opisthotonos; and is a valuable remedy in the treatment of epilepsy when the paroxysms recur periodically. In sleeplessness it is preeminently an effective remedy for those who are suffering from malnutrition, from emaciation, and from blood degeneration, accompanied by extreme exhaustion of the nervous system. Not only is the brain anemic, but the entire body likewise. By keeping a weak and exhausted patient in a prone position both day and night; by the liberal use of a hot liquid diet;

and by the administration of Arsenicum as a restorative medicine, a subtle and charming effect is speedily produced, as is evidenced by pleasant and abundant sleep at night, and the rapid regaining of health and spirits during the daytime.

AURUM

General Action.—Aurum affects the connective tissues, producing degenerations of the bones, glandular organs, and mucous membranes, similar to those found in syphilitic, mercurial, or scrofulous disease. Hyperemia accompanies all other symptoms as a pathological characteristic.

Brain and Spinal Cord.—Tearing headache deep in forehead, with congestion of the brain, and worse from mental work.

Mind.—Has no confidence in himself, and thinks others have none; has a feeling of self-condemnation and worthlesness. Great mental anguish; tired of life, and cannot keep the mind from thoughts of suicide. The melancholia may be of a religious form, when constant prayer may be the most noticeable symptom. The memory is weak, and mental labor is difficult.

Sleep.—Sobs during sleep, or screams aloud from frightful dreams; wakeful during the night, but without lassitude in the morning.

Accompaniments.—Fetid nasal discharge; caries of the bones, especially about the nose and palate; rhinitis; sees things double; boring pain behind the ear; offensive otorrhea; inflammation and degeneration of the liver and kidneys; chronic orchitis, and uterine prolapsus from congestion.

Special Sphere of Action.—Aurum has been considered the remedy in melancholia, and particularly if due to syphilitic disease, or to the abuse of the mercurials; but in our

BAPTISIA

General Action.—It disorganizes the blood, and produces putrid conditions in all parts of the body, with great prostration and exhaustion.

Brain and Spinal Cord.—Cerebral congestion; face has a besotted appearance; dull, heavy pain at the base of the brain; paralysis of the left side, with numbness.

Mind.—Confused as if drunk; feels as if he were sliding away; bed feels too hard (also Arnica); thinks his body is scattered about, and struggles constantly to get himself together; restless, but too lifeless to indulge in active exertion; can be roused, but before answering a question, falls asleep again.

Sleep.—Sleeps well till three A.M. (also Nux Vomica); is then restless till morning; cannot sleep because he thinks his head and body are scattered about; restless, with frightful dreams; mutters in a delirious way even while partially asleep.

Accompaniments.—Intensely fetid breath; dry, hot mouth; tongue very dry and brown, and marked sordes on the teeth; involuntary stools of a strongly offensive nature; the diarrhea is brownish in color, and often looks like decomposed blood.

Special Sphere of Action.—Baptisia may be used in mania and melancholia when there are stupor, rapid and profound degeneration simulating the typhoid state, and when the patient manifests the peculiar mental symptom that he "cannot get himself together". It is a singular fact that many insane patients have the delusion that their bodies are scattered, and they cannot keep themselves in a state of bodily contiguity.

BELLADONNA

General Action.—Belladonna acts upon the cerebrospinal system, causing intense cerebral hyperemia. There is a bright red face, dilated pupils, intolerance of light, and violent spasms of the muscles of the face, neck and arms.

Brain and Spinal Cord.—Severe headache, especially in the frontal region; the headache is of a throbbing nature (also Golonoin and Cactus); the pains come suddenly, and as suddenly depart; fulness of the head, with throbbing arteries; boring, shooting pains in the head, all aggravated by noise.

Mind.—Belladonna develops two distinct states of mind. One where the patient is flushed; the mental powers seem unduly excited and exaggerated. Hallucinations and illusions of sight are present; he sees giant forms; these sometimes excite fear and laughter; and maniacal state in which the patient is merry (also Hyoscyamus); most characteristic there are furious delusions and rage; the patient tears clothing, bites, strikes, kicks, howls, shrieks, and wants to get away. There is a contrary state where the patient passes into a stupid and dazed condition; the pupils remain widely dilated; the eyes are staring and insensible to light; there is heavy stertorous breathing; the face is purplish red; the patient refuses to speak; there is marked rigidity or steady tension of the muscles; and occasionally there is low muttering delirium.

Sleep.—Sleepy, yet cannot sleep (also Gelsemium); jerking of the limbs in sleep; dreams of murder, of robbery, and of danger from fire; sleeplessness from excessive cerebral hyperemia.

Accompaniments.—Spasmodic condition of all the sphincter muscles; paralysis of the left side, with twitching of the muscles of the right side; bright red condition of the skin; active inflammatory condition in the throat, chest, kidneys, bladder, and genital organs.

Special Sphere of Action.—It is particularly useful in conditions of mental excitement in any form of insanity. It is indicated in full-blooded people, with a tendency to cerebral hyperemia in threatened apoplexy, and in insanity following acute diseases. In his mania the patient is likely to be wild, fierce, trying to escape, or to injure those who are in attendance upon him. He manifests a pugnacious disposition which renders him an unpleasant person to care for. His eyes are bright, the conjunctivæ are congested, the pupils are dilated, and the mucous membranes are dry, particularly about the throat. The skin is hot; the face is flushed. Later the patient may become dull and stupid, disinclined to answer questions, and unwilling to be disturbed. Belladonna is also useful in the beginning of meningitis, having an active influence in controlling cerebral hyperemia, and subduing with remarkable efficacy the processes of inflammation.

BRYONIA

General Action.—Serous membranes are especially affected by Bryonia. This drug seems to have marked affinity for pleural coverings of the lungs, and for the peritoneal linings of the abdomen. Again, it affects the joints, producing rheumatic pains; and it likewise pays its respects to the brain and its membranes, producing symptoms of active and intense congestion.

Brain and Spinal Cord.—Head feels confused and full as after a night's dissipation; there is frontal headache extending backward to the occiput (Belladonna, Spigelia, and Gelsemium have headache running from the occiput to the forehead); headache as if the head would burst; this pain grows worse during the day, and is aggravated by motion; head feels too full, and there is much vertigo.

Mind.—Depression and moroseness without cause; the patient is irritable and wishes to be alone (also Coca); is obstinate and passionate, and is troubled with what has been called "pure cussedness" (also Nux Vomica); the patient worries much about business affairs.

Sleep.—Sleep is very restless; during sleep is troubled with somnambulism; sleeplessness from thoughts crowding upon each other; dreams about the business of the day.

Accompaniments.—Cough, usually dry, but sometimes there is sputum which is streaked with blood; cannot take a deep breath; stitching pains in his side, aggravated by motion; sensation as if the head and chest would fall to pieces on coughing; intense thirst for large quantities of water.

Special Sphere of Action.—Characteristics which call for Bryonia are: An apathetic mental condition, ranging from languor to torpor, aggravated by motion of the head. The patient is disposed to be irritable when disturbed or aroused, and the remedy is useful for the bad effects following the manifestations of violence and anger. It is not a remedy on which we rely greatly in the cure of mental disease. It has been of special service in epidemics of influenza or la grippe; in congestions following exposure to cold, and when there has been a tendency to diseased conditions of the serous membranes. It is a useful remedy in constipation occurring among the insane when the stools are large, dark and dry as if burned, and expelled with great difficulty.

CACTUS GRANDIFLORUS

General Action.—This drug appears to have a special affinity for the heart and its nerves, causing more or less irregular action; constricting pain about the heart, with anguish.

Brain and Spinal Cord.—Throbbing pains in the vertex of the head, and along the spine.

Mind.—Melancholia; unconquerable sadness; fear of death (also Aconite); believes his disease incurable (also Ignatia, Lilium Tigrinum, Natrum Muriaticum, and Sepia).

Sleep.—Sleeplessness, with pulsations at the pit of the stomach; palpitation of the heart, and a sensation of palpitation in the top of the head; delirium at night and during sleep, which ceases on awakening (also Gelsemium).

Accompaniments.—Sensation as if an iron band were about the heart, preventing its normal movements; pain in the apex of the heart, shooting down to the fingers of the left hand; irregularity of the heart's action, now rapid and again slow; slow pulse (also Digitalis).

Special Sphere of Action.—Melancholia, particularly in women, with a sensation of constriction about the heart; palpitation of the heart, and a corresponding palpitation on the top of the head.

CALCAREA CARBONICUM

General Action.—This drug seems to have a special affinity for the lymphatic system; its physiological action is not thoroughly understood, but provings and clinical experiences point to the glands of the body as the organs primarily affected.

Brain and Spinal Cord.—It produces a brain fag, frontal headache, with heaviness of the head, worse from reading or writing; it produces chorea, with one-sided movement; and it produces epilepsy, with aura running downward.

Mind.—Forgetfulness; probably one of the most effective remedies for this difficulty; the patient misplaces words (compare Agaricus and Arnica); fears she will lose her reason; that misfortune is impending; that people will observe her confusion of mind; peevishness; anxiety and shrinking on the approach of evening; much mental trouble about imaginary things.

Sleep.—Awakes too early, three A.M.; sleepiness during the daytime; dreams of falling.

Accompaniments.—The menses appear a few days before the proper time, and the flow of blood is often considerable; sensation as if feet and legs were incased in damp stockings; the patient is pale, weak, poorly nourished, and imperfectly developed.

Special Sphere of Action.—The various salts of lime are useful in combating unfortunate constitutional tendencies which are present in the human race, whether sane or insane. Cases of defective growth, either physical or mental, are often improved by the use of Calcarea. It is useful when there is defective bony development, and also when there is emaciation due to constitutional causes. In glandular troubles with lymphatic swellings, it is efficacious in affording relief. The Calcarea patient is of light complexion, of scrofulous appearance, inclined to lay on flabby fat, has a large abdomen, a bulging forehead, and a small neck; the patient is disposed to sweat a good deal about the head, and is troubled with cold feet. Calcarea patients are apt to be apprehensive at times, and to fear that they will go "crazy"; but generally a sluggish and apathetic mental state is present. It is especially adapted to cases of mild but sluggish melancholia in fat, flabby, non-energetic and pot-bellied persons.

CALCAREA-PHOSPHORICUM

General Action.—Similar to the carbonate of lime.

Brain and Spinal Cord.—Cerebral anemia; vertigo, worse on rising; trembling of the limbs.

Mind.—Forgetfulness of what has been done a few moments before; writes wrong words, and the same word twice or more times; wishes to be at home although he is at home; general failure of the mental powers.

Sleep.—Drowsiness all day, yawning and stretching; dreams of past experiences during the night.

Accompaniments.—Pale and flabby conditions, with cold and blue extremities; imperfect circulation; general sluggishness of all the bodily functions.

Special Sphere of Action.—Dementia, especially of young persons and those addicted to masturbation, or those who have exhausted themselves from masturbation; senile dementia, loss of memory from old age, or from cerebral disease.

CAMPHOR

General Action.—It acts upon the cerebro-spinal system, depressing the motor and intellectual centers.

Brain and Spinal Cord.—It produces vertigo and heaviness of the head, constriction of the brain, with throbbing in the cerebrum. Mentally, there is anxiety and extreme restlessness, and a sense of intolerable prostration; from this prostration the mind sometimes rises to great maniacal excitement, somewhat similar to that produced by Veratrum Album.

Accompaniments.—Icy coldness of the whole body; clammy and exhausting sweats; cramps, particularly of the lower limbs; all symptoms are aggravated at night, from motion and from cold.

Special Sphere of Action.—Exhaustion and collapse from mania, from epilepsy, or from melancholia with excitement.

CANNABIS INDICA

General Action.—It acts upon the cerebro-spinal system, producing various effects; sometimes it causes a mild exhilaration, and again it stimulates the prover to intense and exalted ecstacy; it produces decided effects upon the physical system, and stirs the mind to a wonderful variety of action. In this respect it somewhat resembles Opium, Agaricus, Belladonna, and Alcohol.

Brain and Spinal Cord.—Pleasurable intoxication, with bright, shining eyes; heaviness of the arms and legs, making it difficult to move or exercise; a sensation as if the head were opening and shutting along the vertex.

Mind.—Numerous hallucinations and illusions; sensations and motions are greatly exaggerated; time and space seem immeasurable; a few seconds seem to be ages or cycles of time; a few rods seem an immense distance; the patient is unable to recall any thought or event of the past on account of the multitude of images which at present crowd upon the brain; great mental exaltation, with singing and laughing; but this exaltation is followed by sadness, depression and weakness; the natural tendency of the individual is exaggerated under the influence of Cannabis Indica; the mild and gentle persons become more pleasant, happy and agreeable than common, while those possessing irritable dispositions become exceedingly vicious and violent under this drug.

Sleep.—Excessive sleepiness; voluptuous dreams in which are realized the prophesies and promises of Mahomet's heaven for the time being; but morning discovers to the tired dreamer only profuse seminal emission. Dreams of anger, of dead bodies, and of horrible objects; intense nightmare.

Accompaniments.—Frequent micturition, with much burning in the urethra; urine starts slowly and dribbles in a feeble stream; sexual desires greatly increased; violent erections when walking, or riding, or sitting still, and without amorous thoughts, except during the dreams.

Special Sphere of Action.—Nervous diseases, with delusions relating to time and space, accompanied by unusual sexual disturbances, followed by weakness of mind, tremulousness and exhaustion of body. It may be useful in relieving the symptoms of general paresis and catalepsy. The cataleptic state may sometimes be induced by an overpowering belief in the patient's mind that time and space are too vast for change, hence a disinclination to make effort.

CANTHARIS

General Action.—This drug acts upon the cerebro-spinal system, and it affects the genito-urinary tract most positively.

Brain and Spinal Cord.—Cerebral congestions; convulsions resembling hydrophobia, which are produced or aggravated by the sight or sound of water. Hughes denies this symptom, but we have observed some Cantharis cases that were much disturbed by seeing water, or any bright, glistening substance (also Stramonium).

Mind.—Sudden loss of memory; furious delirium; barking like a dog; paroxysms of rage excited by any bright, dazzling object; amorous frenzy; intolerable sexual desire; mania, with a tendency to swear (also Anacardium); violent, contradictory moods; restlessness, culminating in attacks of rage; great activity and sensitiveness of the mind.

Sleep.—Sleeplessness; light sleep with anxious dreams; erections during sleep (also Cannabis Indica), followed by wakefulness and anxiety.

Accompaniments.—Intense burning and smarting pains along the urethra; spasmodic pains in the region of the bladder; paroxysmal pains in both kidneys; the back in the region of the kidneys is sensitive to touch; constant urging to urinate; painful evacuation, drop by drop, of bloody urine, or pure blood; sharp, burning pains in the genital organs, accompanied by erections and fierce desire for sexual intercourse.

Special Sphere of Action.—Cantharis is useful among the insane when the female patient suffers with an intense nymphomania, or the male is afflicted with satyriasis. There is usually an inflammatory condition in some portion of the genito-urinary tract which so excites the sexual desire that the patient loses entirely his self-control, and resorts to the most debasing practices, in order to gratify his insane sexual impulses. The patient has at times a furious delirium, during which he will cry, or bark like a dog, and at times he will manifest great excitement at the sight of water. This latter symptom is suggestive of the conditions present in hydrophobia. (Picric Acid is similar in its action to Cantharis, and in large doses it produces an almost uncontrollable sexual excitement. It is a valuable remedy when sexual excesses have produced exhaustion of the vital forces and a condition of neurasthenia prevails. It is also useful in melancholia with indifference, want of will power, and abject despair. Even in acute dementia with utter exhaustion it is a rival of Phosphoric Acid. There is burning along the spine, weakness of the legs and back, severe pains in the back and occiput, going up to the supraorbital notch. The least exertion causes prostration. In such cases it has proved of striking benefit among the insane).

CAUSTICUM

General Action.—Causticum depresses the function of the motor nerves, especially those which take their origin from neuclei in the medulla oblongata.

Brain and Spinal Cord.—Vertigo, with a tendency to fall either forward or to the side; brought on by motion, or looking steadily at any object. Paralysis of the recti muscles, or of the muscles of the face, tongue, throat, or, more rarely, of the bladder and extremities.

Mind.—Timid, uneasy, fretful; disinclined to work and cannot fix the attention upon any task; the patient is sallow and sickly in appearance; is apprehensive and despondent; distrustful, and as is often the case with an invalid, self-control is partially lost, and he is inclined to break into peevish periods of impotent anger.

Sleep.—Restless; the limbs twitch and jerk, but without interrupting sleep.

Accompaniments.—Weakness of the vocal cords, with catarrhal inflammation of the larynx; hoarseness worse in the morning; painful cough with difficult expectoration of soapy tasting mucus; stiffness of the joints; contraction of the adjacent tendons brought on and aggravated by exposure to cold.

Special Sphere of Action.—Causticum is especially indicated in partial paralysis of the muscles supplied by a single nerve, though it is sometimes prescribed with benefit for the paralysis following cerebral apoplexy; in either case accompanied by irritable mental weakness and indecision. It is a remedy for the constitutionally timid, and for anemic persons of scrofulous habit.

CHAMOMILLA

General Action.—It acts on the cerebro-spinal nervous system, with characteristic affections of the emotional sphere.

Brain and Spinal Cord.—Violent, constricting, pressing, boring headache; pressure from the vertex extending over the forehead and temples; congestion of the brain following fits of anger (also Bryonia); stiffness of the cervical muscles; drawing pains in the scapulæ; pain in the back extending through the abdomen to the front, and into the genitals; severe pain in the loins and hip joints.

Mind.—Irritable, impatient, peevish and snappish; extreme sensitiveness to external impressions (also Coffea, Ignatia, Belladonna and Staphisagria); imagines he hears voices of absent friends at night; bad effects of anger; the patient is extremely cross and sensitive (Nux Vomica is cross, but not so sensitive as Chamomilla).

Sleep.—Sleeplessness from pain, and from ill-temper; even while sleeping the patient moans, weeps, wails, and starts suddenly; on falling asleep is tormented by anxious and frightful dreams.

Accompaniments.—Sharp toothache; gripping colic, with flatulence; severe pains across the abdomen, followed by bilious diarrhoea, and acrid discharges from the vagina.

Special Sphere of Action.—Chamomilla is useful in conditions of excessive hyperesthesia, and this oversensitiveness is accompanied by a corresponding mental state which has been well described as one of "snappish irritability". The patient is cross, impatient, and irritable. Nothing suits him; he is angry, and cannot endure being spoken to, and will not reply respectfully or even decently to any one who addresses him. (Compare Antimonium Tartrate). The patient cannot bear pain, and makes excessive complaint because of slight ailments. This remedy is frequently prescribed for these symptoms among the insane, and is of a great service in affording relief to the oversensitive. It relieves the sleeplessness of those who lie awake on account of severe pain, such as neuralgia affecting a single nerve, or a small group of nerves. Such patients are exceedingly cross and irritable, and indulge in frequent jerkings of the limbs, and twitchings of groups of muscles. It is a remedy that has acquired much fame on account of its success in relieving the sleeplessness of children, and of weak and nervous women.

CHINA

General Action.—China acts upon the ganglionic nervous system, and hence it affects especially the functions of vegetative life. China changes both the quantity and the quality of the blood. Under its influence the blood becomes more fluid than normal; the circulation becomes impaired, and we have general debility and erethism, followed by chills, fever, sweat, and finally hemorrhages. China produces congestion of the liver, obstructing the function of that organ; it produces excessive sensitiveness of the entire nervous system.

Brain and Spinal Cord.—Intense congestion of the brain; intense throbbing headache; vertigo; ringing in the ears; deafness; blindness. With the dizziness there is a feeling as if the head would burst. This feeling is worse from motion or sudden anger; insupportable pain in small of back, like a cramp, worse from least movement.

Mind.—Chooses wrong words, and makes feeble and senseless expressions. The patient cherishes a fixed idea that he is unhappy, and that he is persecuted by his enemies;

feels impelled to jump out of bed; wants to destroy himself, but lacks courage; is low-spirited, gloomy, and has no desire to live; cherishes an uncontrollable anxiety; and, above all, is stubborn and disobedient. Patients are sometimes sent to insane asylums because they have been made insane, in my opinion, not alone by the diseases from which they suffered, but also by a blind, reckless and unwarrantable use of Cinchona, or its alkaloids, given in overpowering and disastrous doses. Cinchona, if unwisely used, may become as dangerous in its effects as the excessive use of alcoholic stimulants.

Sleep.—Irresistible desire to sleep after eating; constant yet unrefreshing sleep; or at times sleepless from ideas crowding too rapidly upon each other (also Apis and Coffea). The patient is bent upon making plans for the future, hence his sleep is short and unrefreshing.

Accompaniment.—Loss of appetite; slow digestion; thin, watery; involuntary diarrhea; weakness and disability from long continued sickness, and from excessive losses of fluid from the body; fever recurring at somewhat regular intervals.

Special Sphere of Action.—Melancholia and subacute mania when there are general anemia, profound debility, and tendency to periodical aggravation of all the symptoms.

CICUTA VIROSA

General Action.—This drug is a cerebro-spinal irritant, producing epileptiform convulsions, tetanus, and generally tonic and clonic spasms.

Brain and Spinal Cord.—Severe occipital headache; vertigo, with opisthotonos.

Mind.—Dull and stupid, or the patient indulges in weeping and howling; sometimes great mental excitement exists and the patient sings, shouts, and dances.

Accompaniments.—Grinding of teeth; swelling of tongue; difficulty in speech; involuntary twitching of muscles in the arms and fingers (also Cuprum).

Special Sphere of Action.—Mental depression and anxiety, accompanied by vertigo, after traumatism; general paralysis, with spasmodic twitchings; sometimes loss of consciousness; mental anxiety, with violent hiccough. Cicuta is one of the most effective remedies for persistent hiccoughing known in the Materia Medica.

CIMICIFUGA (Actea Racemosa)

General Action.—It produces cerebral and spinal hyperemia, with irregularity of motion, and great weakness and tremulousness of the extremities.

Brain and Spinal Cord.—Headache throughout the whole brain, with sense of soreness in the occipital region; vertigo; brain feels too heavy and too large for the cranium; the top of the head feels as if it would fly off.

Mind.—Great melancholy, with sleeplessness, followed sometimes by transient exhilaration; hallucinations of sight, sees rats, sheep, etc.; sensation as if a heavy black cloud had settled over her, and enveloped her head, so that all was darkness and confusion; at the same time there seems to be a weight like lead upon the heart; suspicious, indifferent; taciturn; takes no interest in household matters (also Sepia).

Sleep.—Sleeplessness from nervous irritation; sleeplessness, with great depression and despair.

Accompaniments.—There is a general rheumatic diathesis; severe cutting pains in the joints and in the back; in women there is with the mental depression a sense of weight and bearing down in the uterine region (also Belladonna), with a feeling of heaviness and torpor in the lower extremities, retarded menstruation; suppression of menses from a cold, with rheumatic pains in the head, extending down to the neck and back; tremulousness of the muscles throughout the body.

Special Sphere of Action.—Mental depression associated with uterine diseases; mental depression accompanied by rheumatic pains; mental depression and tremulousness, following overwork and active dissipation; delirium tremens; bad effects of opium. It is indicated in general paresis when the patient is weak and exceedingly tremulous throughout the whole body, and particularly in the melancholic stage of the disease.

COCCULUS

General Action.—On the motor tract of the cerebrospinal axis, and especially on the cerebellum, producing fulness of the head, and a swaying of the body in a semi-circular direction, with loss of power in the lower limbs.

Brain and Spinal Cord.—Vertigo, with inclination to vomit; sensation as if the head were swollen; headache in the occiput and nape of neck; sensation as if the back of head were opening and shutting like a door; headache aggravated by riding in a wagon; paralytic weakness of the back and legs, and a feeling as if soles of the feet were asleep.

Mind.—Vacillating; cannot accomplish any work; slowness of apprehension; time passes too quickly (too slowly, Cannabis Indica); sobbing, moaning and groaning; thoughts continue upon some one unpleasant subject; depressed; easily offended; every trifle makes him angry; a delusion that his organs are hollow; sometimes this delusion relates to the head, or the chest, or the abdomen.

Sleep.—Sleeplessness from night-watching (Colchicum); sleep aggravates all the symptoms (Lachesis).

Accompaniments.—Physical and mental symptoms aggravated by eating or drinking; intense nausea; an inclination to vomit while riding in a carriage or a boat; great distension of the abdomen, with colic; in a female, cramping pains in the uterus and ovaries, with nausea and headache; violent spasmodic pains during the menstrual flux, after mortification or disappointment.

Special Sphere of Action.—Diseases accompanied by intense vertigo, relieved by lying down; diseases caused by overexertion, overstudy, overdrinking; the motion of travel; uterine disorders at the change of life; victims of masturbation; victims of excessive ambition who have been disappointed, snubbed, and angered by those around them. (For dissipation and disappointment we also think of Nux Vomica, of Gelsemium, and of Ignatia).

COFFEA CRUDA

General Action.—Acts upon the cerebro-spinal system, causing an increased susceptibility to external impressions—that is, a general hyperesthesia of the nervous system.

Brain and Spinal Cord.—Headache from thinking; headache as if the head were torn or dashed to pieces; headache as if a nail were driven into the head (also Hepar Sulphur and Ignatia); a Coffea headache, like Nux Vomica, is worse after eating.

Mind.—Ecstasy; full of ideas; quick to act; great mental restlessness; all the senses under Coffea are stirred to acute and rapid action; under its primary and secondary influences the mind oscillates between the heights of ecstatic and sensitive joy, and the depths of gloomiest and most dismal despair.

Sleep.—Sleeplessness because mind is very active (also

China), and because the emotions have been driven by pleasant occurrences into a state of excessive excitement.

Accompaniments.—General acuteness of the senses; distressing and insupportable pains, particularly neuralgia of the right side of the face and head; an aversion to the open air because it seems to aggravate the pain.

Special Sphere of Action.—Melancholia with excitement and sleeplessness; hysterical affections produced by excessive pleasurable emotions.

COLCHICUM

General Action.—It acts upon the processes of nutrition; increases the secretions generally, and especially the quantity of urea and uric acid eliminated. In poisonous doses it is an irritant to the alimentary tract, and causes death by collapse and paralysis of respiration.

Brain and Spinal Cord.—Boring headache over the eyes; pressure, especially in the occiput; paralytic sensations and numbness of the hands and feet.

Mind.—Sensitive to external impressions, especially bright lights and strong odors; memory weak; intellect clouded; the patient is peevish; fretful, and never satisfied.

Sleep.—Sleeplessness after night-watching or studying at night; awakened from sleep by dreadful dreams.

Accompaniments.—Great thirst, but no appetite; aversion to food, and especially to the smell of food; great distension of the abdomen, with colicky pains; dark and scanty urine; rheumatism, accompanied by great exhaustion, and by weakness of both body and mind. The pains are all of a boring nature.

Special Sphere of Action.—It acts well in patients who are depressed and irritable, and who are of a rheumatic or gouty diathesis.

COLOCYNTH

General Action.—This drug acts upon the ganglionic nervous system, more particularly upon the solar plexus, the lumbar and the femoral nerves, and the tissues which these nerves supply.

Brain and Spinal Cord.—Pressive frontal headache, tearing and digging through the whole brain; sharp, cutting pains along the tracts of the main nerves leading from the brain; cramping pains in the lumbar region, extending down to the legs, especially along the course of the sciatic nerve.

Mind.—Extremely irritable and easily angered; impatient and morose. In mental irritability, Colocynth imitates Chamomilla and Nux Vomica.

Sleep.—Sleeplessness on account of acute cramping pains; inclined to sleep as soon as the pains pass away.

Accompaniments.—Sharp, colicky pains in the abdomen, doubling the victim up like a jack-knife; diarrhea watery, yellow, frothy, and accompanied by much flatulence.

Special Sphere of Action.—Persons of nervo-bilious temperament, and those suffering from severe cramping and neuralgic pains, and from the effects of sudden outbursts of anger (Bryonia).

CONIUM-MACULATUM

General Action.—Its effects are especially noticeable upon the motor nervous tract; it produces paralysis from the feet up. One of the best provings of hemlock may be found in the death of Socrates.

Brain and Spinal Cord.—Intense vertigo, worse on lying down; headache as if the head would burst; pain in the occiput, and at each heart beat the brain at the base feels as if stabbed with a sharp knife; trembling of limbs; sensation of weakness in the back and limbs; sense of exhaustion as if paralysed.

Mind.—Loss of memory; inability to make any mental effort.

Sleep.—Unrefreshing, and disturbed by frightful dreams.

Accompaniments.—Palpitation of the heart; violent, spasmodic, dry cough; sexual desire without erection.

Special Sphere of Action.—Senile dementia; mental weakness; loss of memory; peevishness; vertigo. It is useful when persons suffer from the ill effects of ungratified sexual desire; it is therefore useful in relieving the ailments of old maids, of widows, of widowers, of old people generally, and of those who have a tendency to paralysis, especially in the lower limbs; likewise for children who appear to be prematurely old.

CUPRUM METALLICUM

General Action.—In massive doses it produces nausea, purging, and collapse. Its action upon the nervous system, detailed below, is secondary, and follows its continued administration in smaller quantities.

Brain and Spinal Cord.—Irritation of the cerebro-spinal axis, with painful spasmodic contractions of the abdominal muscles, and those of the lower extremities; or clonic convulsions not limited to any single part, accompanied by loss of consciousness, and followed by a deep sleep.

Mind.—Violent; delirium, with great fear; shrinks from any one who approaches (also Stramonium); or bites, strikes, and tears to pieces everything within reach, as does Belladonna. In lesser degree there may be restlessness and melancholy, with a constant sense of approaching misfortune.

Sleep.—Very heavy; almost a comatose condition, or intensely sleepy, and unable to rest.

Accompaniments.—Spasmodic attacks of dyspnea; chest feels contracted, almost to suffocation; ineffectual efforts to vomit, with contractive pains in the stomach at intervals.

Special Sphere of Action.—In some cases of idiopathic epilepsy it has seemed to be of service, but is most useful in the spasmodic cramps in weak, nervous individuals; those in whom mental or physical overwork has advanced to complete exhaustion. Reaction is deficient, and relapse follows the slightest indiscretion, until Cuprum starts the patient on the way to recovery.

DIGITALIS

General Action.—Acts upon the cerebro-spinal system, especially affecting the cardiac branch of the pneumogastric nerve. The first effect upon the heart is to strengthen the contractions and diminish the number of heart beats; the force of these contractions being increased, exhaustion soon follows; then the number of beats becomes greatly increased, with a marked decrease in their strength; this loss of strength may continue until paralysis results.

Brain and Spinal Cord.—Headache, with congestion; marked pulsations in the forehead (Cactus has pulsations in the top of the head); heavy, paralyzed feelings in the legs.

Mind.—Anxiety, and fear of the future; low spirits, with inclination to weep; the eyes seem constantly floating in tears; anxiety as from a troubled conscience; fear of death; fear that the heart will stop beating.

Sleep.—Uneasy, unrefreshing sleep; frequently startled, and awakes easily many times during the night (also Phosphorus).

Accompaniments.—Constant urging to urinate; the urine is scanty, coffee-colored, and has a brick-dust sediment (also

Lycopodium); extremely weak and rapid pulse, or a slow, full, sluggish pulse.

Special Sphere of Action.—Melancholia following masturbation; mental depression in cases of heart disease; insanity when the circulation is weak and greatly disturbed.

FERRUM METALLICUM

General Action.—This drug produces marked changes in the condition of the blood; under its influence the number of red corpuscles is diminished; the watery portions of the blood are increased, while the albumen is decreased; it produces a condition which Dr. S. Weir Mitchell has described as "fat anemia". The patients are weak, pale, and anemic, yet an appearance of flabby fulness sometimes remains.

Brain and Spinal Cord.—Congestions of the brain, with sense of fulness, and throbbing pains in the head (also Glonoin), worse after midnight; a feeling of paralysis in the lower limbs.

Mind.—Muddled and confused; depression of spirits in women, especially at the menstrual period; anxiety and peevishness; the slightest contradiction angers (also Chamomilla).

Sleep.—Sleepy, but unable to sleep (also Belladonna and Gelsemium); feels sleepy usually as a result of debility; wakens frequently during the night (also Phosphorus); and feels weary, prostrated and unrefreshed in the morning (also Nux Vomica).

Accompaniments.—General weakness and prostration; face pale, but flushes easily; sometimes there is emaciation, at other times the fat remains, but in all cases there is great weakness; peculiar pallor of the countenance, menses too early and too profuse; diarrhea of hot, undigested stools;

while the patient is pale when quiet, the least excitement or motion produces rosy cheeks.

Special Sphere of Action.—Hypochondriacal melancholia; weak and chlorotic women; children who are badly nourished, and prone to diarrhea. The form of iron from which we have obtained the best results has been the citrate.

GELSEMIUM

General Action.—It paralyzes the respiratory center in the medulla, and the motor nerves generally, especially those of the eye. Under its influence there is a passive venous congestion.

Brain and Spinal Cord.—Passive venous congestion of the cerebrum; brain feels bruised; great heaviness of the head; dull, dragging pains in the occiput; scalp feels sore (also Arnica, Bryonia and Nux Vomica); giddiness; drawing, contracting pains in the calves of the legs; paralysis of the muscles of motion.

Mind.—Dull and stupid; the victim feels as if grossly intoxicated; unable to think or fix the attention; fear of death, with moderate anxiety concerning the present.

Sleep.—Drowsy, but cannot sleep; as soon as he falls asleep he becomes delirious and mutters while dreaming (also Cactus); sleeplessness, with a wide-awake but helpless feeling.

Accompaniments.—Prostration of the whole muscular system; shooting, tearing, neuralgic pains along the tracks of the large nerves; rapid and irregular action of the heart; chilliness, followed by fever and stupidity.

Special Sphere of Action.—Mental depression resulting from fright, from bad or exciting news, or from anticipation of coming trouble, as when a student contemplates the horrors of final examination, Neuralgia; convulsions; paralysis; epilepsy; hysteria; rheumatic congestions; dysmenorrhea; and cerebro-spinal meningitis. Gelsemium is especially applicable to young and nervous people. It relieves sleeplessness in recent or incipient drunkards; in brain workers, in business men, and in those who have become suddenly exhausted by work or worry, or both. The Gelsemium patients present a heavy and besotted appearance. They are dull and stupid, and seem to be on the verge of heavy slumber, yet cannot sleep.

GLONOIN

General Action.—It dilates the arterial system, increases the fulness and rapidity of the pulse, and produces accelerated respiration, paralysis, loss of reflex action and sensation, and death from stoppage of respiration.

Brain and Spinal Cord.—Head feels full to bursting, with violent throbbing, usually without severe pain, except when shaking the head; with slight motion sharp violent pains shoot through the brain (also Bryonia); the skull seems too small, and feels as if it would burst with every beat of the heart.

Mind.—Ideas become confused; loses his way on familiar streets; does not recognize them; falls down, with loss of consciousness.

Sleep.—Restless sleep, with confused dreams, yet difficult to awaken.

Accompaniments.—The whole action of Glonoin centers about its power to produce sudden and violent changes in the circulation. It is characterized by a full strong pulse; the arteries throbbing visibly as under Belladonna; and active congestions are seen in the hot, bright red skin which almost immediately follows its administration.

Special Sphere of Action.—This remedy fits very

HEPAR SULPHUR

General Action.—This drug produces enlargement and suppuration of the lymphatic glands, an unhealthy skin, ulcers, eczematous eruptions, and catarrhal conditions of the mucous membranes.

Brain and Spinal Cord.—Pain on one side of the head as if a plug or dull nail were driven into the brain (Ignatia and Coffea); a sense of swashing in the brain.

Mind.—Low-spirited and irritable; memory weak; he forgets words and places; dwells on former unpleasant incidents which make him feel discouraged (also Natrum Muriaticum); is even suicidal. The anxiety is greatest in the evening.

Sleep.—Violent starts when falling asleep; excess of thoughts keep him awake in the latter half of the night.

Accompaniments.—Profuse mucous secretions, with sharp splinter-like pains; great sensitiveness of all affected parts; cannot bear any pressure. The symptoms are all better with warmth, and made worse by exposure to cold.

Special Sphere of Action.—Hepar Sulphur is one of the remedies less used among the insane for the direct control of mental symptoms than for the improvement of their physical state. Many other remedies have similar symptoms, but none other takes its place in the management and prevention of suppurative processes. It is also particularly indicated in the atonic dyspepsias, with a craving for stimulants and condiments.

HYOSCYAMUS

General Action.—It produces special effects upon the sensorium, causing hallucinations of sight, and great mental activity. In large doses, it produces a temporary paralysis of the voluntary muscles, with partial obliteration of consciousness.

Brain and Spinal Cord.—Cerebral congestion of a milder type than that produced by Belladonna; trembling of the limbs; spasmodic twitchings of the muscles of the back, and in the organs of locomotion.

Mind.—Delirium, accompanied by periods of stupor; thinks he is in the wrong place; foolish laughter; almost always jolly; talks in a hurried and cheerful manner; intensely jealous; at times lascivious; inclined to uncover the body and expose the sexual organs; sings amorous and obscene songs.

Sleep.—Sleeplessness from excessive mental excitement (also Bryonia and Coffea); sleepless without any apparent cause; dreams of obscene things; has dreams of a terrifying nature, and awakens with a loud scream.

Accompaniments.—Retention of urine (also Cantharis and Arsenicum); sometimes has involuntary discharges of urine (also Causticum); attacks of hiccough (also Ignatia and Cicuta Virosa); spasmodic twitchings in various muscles; tendency to convulsions; dry and spasmodic cough; involuntary stools.

Special Sphere of Action.—It is especially adapted to women who become insane during pregnancy or after parturition; to those who suffer from jealousy or unhappy love; to victims of delirium tremens; and to young people and children who are inclined to convulsive attacks, to epilepsy, and to chorea. In general paresis it is frequently called for to control the delusions. This drug has been famous as a sleep producer for many years. Hyoscyamine and Hyoscine, the active principles of the original drug, have been much experimented with, and perhaps have been used in too large and too frequently repeated doses to secure the best and most satisfactory results. The Hyoscyamus patient is sleepless without apparent cause, save that the nervous system has become somewhat depleted, while at the same time the mind of the patient has been overworn by too long continued or too active use. The Hyoscyamus patient has neither the anxiety of Aconite, the rage of Belladonna, nor the stupidity of Gelsemium, but he displays the individual characteristic of a jolly and wakeful delirium. Hyoscyamus paints the mental tone of its victim a brilliant and luminous red, and stimulates him to sing, in merriest and most vociferous tones, the songs of Venus and Bacchus combined.

HYPERICUM

General Action.—It acts upon the cerebro-spinal system, producing cerebral and spinal hyperemia, with great sensitiveness of the nerves.

Brain and Spinal Cord.—Headache; confusion; vertigo and heaviness; congestion of the spinal cord; convulsions from a blow on the head.

Mind.—Irritable; inclined to speak sharply; sees spirits and spectres; suffers from loss of memory; intense depression after nerve injuries.

Sleep.—Spasmodic jerkings of the limbs on going to sleep; dreams of travelling.

Accompaniments.—Tympanitic distention of the abdomen; great sensitiveness to external impressions.

Special Sphere of Action.—Mental depression following all nerve injuries; convulsions, spinal affections and lockjaw following wounds of the nerves. Hypericum is said to be the Arnica of the nervous system, and in some cases this drug has seemed to have the power of arresting nerve degeneration, notably in one case of progressive muscular atrophy.

IGNATIA

General Action.—It acts upon the cerebro-spinal nervous system, more especially on the spine, producing hyperesthesia of all the senses.

Brain and Spinal Cord.—Congestive headache, following anger or grief, especially grief; headache, with bruised feeling, or a sensation as if a nail were driven in the temples; occipital headache, better from pressure. Its effects upon the spine are shown by the sudden jerkings of the limbs, by twitchings of groups of muscles, by a feeling of heaviness in the feet, with a sensation of burning in the soles of the feet.

Mind.—Intense though partially suppressed grief; anxiety as if crime had been committed; grief following the loss of friends; grief of children after being reproved or punished by parents; fearfulness; irresoluteness; timidity; sad, quiet, melancholy. Sometimes the Ignatia case is hysterical and hilarious temporarily; but soon subsides, and "weeps tears inwardly".

Sleep.—Very light sleep; jerking of the limbs on going to sleep; dreams of one thing particularly of the object of affection.

Accompaniments.—Frequent sighing; desire to take a deep breath; sensitive spine; sharp, constricting pains in the anus; constipation; stools large and soft, but passed with difficulty; spasmodic cough from mental anxiety.

Special Sphere of Action.—Ignatia is a remedy of great value in conditions of profound mental depression, and the cases of melancholia in which it does not find a place during some period of their treatment are very few. It is particularly useful in ailments resulting from grief, the loss of friends, and bad news of any sort; the effects of disappointed love; ailments of a nature which lead to concealment rather than publicity, and over which the patient broods in silence, with sad countenance, and frequent sighing; griefs and troubles about which the patient can rarely be induced to talk, but from which he suffers often to the extent of unhinging his reason, and driving him to despair, and possibly to suicide. It is curative in long continued but suppressed sadness occasioned by family afflictions or by financial misfortunes; in chorea or epilepsy in children whose troubles are occasioned by feeling that they have been unkindly or harshly treated. In general paresis it relieves when there is long continued depression of mind with inclination to mourn and brood over the past, while he also cherishes dark apprehensions relative to the future. The Ignatia patient not only broods and mourns, but likewise has attacks of general restlessness, when he wrings his hands and trembles a good deal. It is useful in hysterical affections when there appears to be great sensitiveness to external impressions, alternate laughing and crying, cold extremities accompanied or followed by the passage of large quantities of pale urine. (Also Gelsemium and Phosphoric Acid). There is severe pain in the head of the character known as *clavus hystericus*. This remedy alone has proven curative in numerous cases of melancholia, particularly for women, where it seems to do better than for men. With men, Arsenicum or Nux Vomica appears to act better.

IODINE

General Action.—Its action through the sympathetic nervous system is upon the glandular organs, in the first instance stimulating their functions, and increasing their secretions; and secondarily, producing atony and advanced or complete atrophy.

Brain and Spinal Cord.—Headache as if a band were drawn tightly around the head; worse with active exertion, as walking rapidly; sometimes a feeling of paralytic weakness in the arms; vertigo on the left side only.

Mind.—Restless; constantly moving about; changes his seat frequently; overcareful; fears an unfavorable outcome to every little occurrence (compare Calcarea Carbonica and Arsenicum); shrinking and fear when any one comes near; low-spirited; irritable and sensitive, especially during digestion. The patient may feel that the brain is stirred up, and that he must keep in constant motion, or go insane.

Sleep.—Restless after midnight, with vivid, anxious dreams; feels constantly as if she had forgotten something.

Accompaniments.—Hoarseness or complete aphonia, with dry croupy cough or wheezing respiration, pulmonary congestion; chronic diarrhea, with bloody mucous stools; enlargement of the thyroid gland, especially if soft, with swelling of the other glands of the neck.

Special Sphere of Action.—Iodine is most successful in elderly persons, with dark hair and eyes, and with a tendency to rapid emaciation. It is indicated in the melancholia of the aged, and in those weakened by the scrofulous diathesis, or succumbing to cretinic conditions. Its remarkable power in resolving and dissipating morbid hypertrophies and cellular new growths renders it, especially in combination with Potassium, of prime service in the organic insanities brought about by the lesions or tertiary syphilis in the central nervous system.

LACHESIS

General Action.—This drug acts upon the blood, and produces decomposition and defibrination of that fluid; consequently Lachesis induces hemorrhages, abscesses, malignant inflammation, gangrene, and pyemia. Upon the nervous system it produces two characteristics: hyperesthesia and intolerance to pressure in all parts of the body, and the aggravation of all symptoms after sleep.

Brain and Spinal Cord.—Intense pressive headache, extending from the frontal region to the base of the brain and to the nose; the headache is accompanied by nausea and vertigo on waking in the morning; there is great weakness in the arms and legs; with the weakness and exhaustion there is sensitiveness to all external impressions, and the slightest constriction around the neck or chest or waist is unbearable.

Mind.—Mental activity, with a tendency to talk much; yet the mind is weak and erratic, and the victim makes many mistakes if he attempts any intellectual work; lack of mental continuity; constantly changing from the one subject to another; jealousy; hallucinations of frightful images. The Lachesis patient thinks himself under superhuman control; also thinks himself dead, and that preparations are being made for a gaudy funeral.

Sleep.—Wide awake in the evening; restless sleep, disturbed by dreams; tossing about in sleep; great sleepiness, but unable to sleep (also Belladonna and Chamomilla).

Accompaniments.—Dimness of vision, with black spots before the eyes; left-sided tonsillitis; difficulty in swallowing liquids; sensitiveness of throat; sensitiveness of internal organs, as well as senitiveness upon the surface of the body; scanty and feeble menses, with dark, bloody discharges; extreme sensitiveness of the uterus, particularly at the menstrual flux and during the climacteric period; general left-sided pains, with great sensitiveness.

Special Sphere of Action.—It is particularly serviceable in the mental depressions which sometimes occur in women at the climacteric period; the patient is often loquacious, and jumps from one subject to another in conversation. It seems to be useful in certain cases of neurasthenia, where it aids in arousing the patient from an apathetic or indifferent condition, and giving him his first start toward recovery. It is called for in insanity following fevers of a low type, and left-sided paralysis (also Arnica and Lycopodium).

LILIUM TIGRINUM

General Action.—It acts upon the heart and causes cardiac irritability, with palpitation. It also produces venous congestions, most pronounced in the female generative organs.

Brain and Spinal Cord.—Dull headache over the left eye, or alternating from side to side; fulness of the head, as if its contents would be pushed out at every aperture; heat in the top of the head; vertigo, which is better in cool air; the whole body feels sore as if pounded (also Arnica and Eupatorium Perfoliatum).

Mind.—Great fear, and dread of insanity (also Sepia and Calcarea Carbonica); fear that should she become insane no one would care for her; loss of memory; uses wrong words; desire to do something with hurried manner, but unable to accomplish anything. Sometimes from depression and anxiety the Lilium patients pass into a mental state where they become peevish and fretful, and where they are inclined to curse and talk in an obscene manner.

Sleep.—Inability to sleep, worse before midnight, restless sleep, and wild feelings in the head; frightful dreams; everything seems hot, particularly in the region of the genitals; twitchings of the legs on falling asleep.

Accompaniments.—Menses too late and scanty; bearing down in the uterine region, with a feeling as if everything were coming out (also Sepia and Belladonna); functional disease of the left ovary, accompanied by stinging, cutting, grasping pains; heart feels as if squeezed by a vise, and as if the blood had been all pressed out.

Special Sphere of Action.—Melancholia with excitement, preceded by ovarian and uterine diseases, and by functional disturbances of the heart; mental disturbances following subinvolution of the uterus; depression of mind after severe and exhausting labors.

LYCOPODIUM

General Action.—This drug acts upon the vegetative system, producing weakness of its powers, and wasting and decay of the tissues. It acts also upon the liver and the digestive tract in such a way as to cause hepatic congestions, constipation, indigestion, and marked accumulations of flatulence.

Brain and Spinal Cord.—Pressing frontal headache, especially right side of the head (Lachesis headache is on the left side); the Lycopodium headache is worse from 4 to 8 P.M.; pressive headache in the vertex (Cactus has throbbing in the vertex); under Lycopodium the hair becomes gray too early in life; it induces falling out of the hair and causes baldness; burning pains between the scapulæ; pain in the small of the back; drawing, tearing pains in all the limbs; stiffness and painfulness of the joints; cramps in the calves of the legs; sensation as if a tight band were bound around the body at the umbilicus; sensation of a band about the head (also Mercurius).

Mind.—Great depression of spirits; very sad, desponding and anxious; doubts about salvation (also Sulphur and Veratrum); weakness of memory, with confusion of thoughts; when the digestive organs are much disturbed, the patient is fretful, irritable and morose, or he may become vehement and angry if crossed in his purpose or desires; at times is imperious and domineering in manner; thinks himself of much importance (also Belladonna, Cuprum, Platina, and Veratrum).

Sleep.—Sleepy during the daytime, wakeful at night, sleep restless; cries and starts in sleep (also Chamomilla and Antimonium Crudum); unrefreshing sleep; feels *blasé* in the morning (also Nux Vomica).

Accompaniments.—Fulness and distention of the abdomen, with flatulence; frequent eructations; variable appetite; considerable hunger, but a small quantity of food produces sensations of fulness (also Cinchona and Sepia); red sediment in the urine (also Digitalis); general aggravation from 4 to 8 P.M.

Special Sphere of Action.—Melancholia accompanied by dyspepsia, flatulence and constipation; subacute mania, with indigestion, chronic hepatitis, and catarrh of the bladder, and chronic rheumatism; mental disturbance in the latter stages of phthisis pulmonalis; emaciation from lack of power to assimilate food, and accompanied by night sweats.

MERCURIUS

General Action.—Acts upon the entire organism, but especially upon the vegetative system, producing depressions of functional power, and decomposing and disintegrating the organic constituents of the body; scretions and excretions are increased, but the secretions become thinner than normal, and the excretions become acrid and excoriating.

Brain and Spinal Cord.—Congestion of the brain, with feeling of a band about the head (also Lycopodium); the scalp is painful to the touch (also Nitric Acid, China, Nux

Vomica and Arnica); weakness and trembling in the limbs and back, worse at night; cold extremities.

Mind.—Great weakness of memory; loss of sense of decency; delusions concerning food; eyes dull and staring; under the influence of impaired vision he becomes suspicious and distrustful of those about him.

Sleep.—Sleepy during the daytime, but sleepless at night, because all pains in the Mercurius patient are aggravated at night.

Accompaniments.—Pale face; swollen tongue and gums; loss of teeth; profuse, watery discharges from the mouth; a sluggish condition of the abdominal organs; foul breath; pain and soreness of all the muscles; bone pains at night and in damp weather.

Special Sphere of Action.—The various mercurial preparations are frequently of use in the treatment of demented or depressed conditions, following scrofulous, syphilitic, rheumatic, and catarrhal affections. The constitution seems to be deeply affected; the blood is impoverished, and the body wastes. There is frequently hectic fever; the skin ulcerates easily; the patient is sleepless, and troubled with twitchings of the limbs and the characteristic Mercurial tremor. In general paresis it is indicated when there is a general heavy and soggy condition of the system; the patient is inclined to be filthy in body and groveling mentally, and inclined to rambling incoherence or apathetic dementia. Experience seems to teach that Mercurius acts better in acute cases when preceded by a few doses of Aconite. It is a drug whose general action covers those mental states which naturally follow disorganization of the physical system by diseases which are the result of exposure to the worst types of both weather and women.

NATRUM MURIATICUM

General Action.—It acts upon the vegetative system, upon the blood, upon the digestive tract, and upon the spleen. Normally, salt is present in every tissue of the body, and this is not to be wondered at, for we use it in almost every article of food. When taken in excess it is highly irritative and disorganizing in its action, and leaves no organ unaffected. Soldiers, sailors and Arctic explorers, and all who are obliged to live upon very salt food, eventually have catarrhal discharges from all the mucous surfaces; thence they pass into a condition known as scurvy; the body emaciates, the blood becomes thinned and is defibrinated; and the bones themselves become tender and brittle.

Brain and Spinal Cord.—Pulsating headache in the vertex every morning; stupefying headache, with nausea; the headache recurs every day at a certain hour; the hair falls out, and the scalp becomes sensitive; there is pain in the small of the back, as if broken; the limbs are weak, trembling, and paralytic.

Mind.—Sadness and depression of spirits, aggravated by sympathy; aversion to men (a very abnormal feminine symptom); profuse weeping followed by loss of memory; difficulty in grasping and retaining one's thoughts.

Sleep.—Falls asleep late at night, and awakens early in the morning; uneasy, anxious sleep; the patient sobs and cries even while sleeping.

Accompaniments.—Blisters on the lips; violent, unquenchable thirst; emaciation, even with an enormous appetite; copious discharges of light urine.

Special Sphere of Action.—Melancholia following intermittent fevers, especially those cases which have been overdosed with quinine; mental impairment in young persons who have suffered with imperfect development and from scorbutic affections; mental depression in girls affected with chlorosis, or profuse leucorrhea; mental diseases of an intermittent type.

NITRIC ACID

General Action.—Nitric Acid, whether applied locally or administered internally, is destructive in its action. Its effects are seen in the blood, glands, bones, skin, mucous membranes, and most characteristically at the various muco-cutaneous junctions, as the mouth or anus.

Brain and Spinal Cord.—Rush of blood to the head; pulsating headache as if the head were tightly bound up as in a vise (compare Antimonium Tartaricum, Gelsemium, and Mercurius).

Mind.—Discontented, and inclined to weep violently; despondent moods; easily discouraged or irritated, and vexed by little things unworthy of notice; anxious about himself; mental work is difficult and distasteful.

Sleep.—Wakens too early in the morning; disturbed by dreams of crimes, dangers, or death.

Accompaniments.—Ragged, unhealthy ulcers, with thin, excoriating, ichorous discharge; thin, irritating nasal catarrh; pains in all parts of the body, as though a splinter or piece of glass were sticking in the flesh; offensive green, undigested diarrhea passed with much straining.

Special Sphere of Action.—This is a deep acting constitutional remedy best indicated in scrawny, thin, dark-skinned persons debilitated by the action of some violent dyscrasia, usually of protracted duration. It is useful in the secondary stage of syphilis, especially in an excessive remedy for the despondency, mental weakness, and irritability which attend profound physical disease.

NUX VOMICA

General Action.—It acts especially upon the spinal cord, causing an excitability of both motor and sensory centers; it produces tetanic convulsions and rigid flexions of the body, such as opisthotonous; it also produces spasmodic contractions of the muscles of the throat, of the face, and of the intestinal and urinary tracts.

Brain and Spinal Cord.—It produces congestion of the brain, and stupefaction. This drug produces a feeling as if the victim had indulged for a long time in a heavy debauch; there is a dull, heavy pain throughout the head, and especially over the left eye or in the occiput; there are spasms of the muscles on the neck, back and limbs, sometimes so severe that the patient stands upon his head and heels with body curved upward.

Mind.—Intense irritability; disposition to find fault with everything; quarrelsome; vindictive, ill-humored (also Bryonia); oversensitive to external impressions; cannot tolerate light or noise (also Belladonna), music or strong odor; inclination to kill beloved friends; inclined to commit suicide, but too cowardly to consummate his desires; extreme sensitiveness to the words and attention of others.

Sleep.—After long continued mental exertion, the Nux Vomica patient is sleepless from an inability to compose the mind and disengage himself from attention to the business he has had in hand; falls asleep late at night; wakens at three A.M., lies awake tossing and fretting for two or three hours, falls asleep when he should get up, and after a short morning nap awakens unrefreshed and ill tempered, his anger rising against himself and those around him.

Accompaniments.—Photophobia, aggravated in the morning; nose plugged with mucus on awakening, followed by profuse watery discharges after the nostrils are relieved of the plug; besotted expression of the face; bitter eructations, with nausea in the morning; pressure and pain in the stomach after eating; constipation with ineffectual urging.

Special Sphere of Action.—This remedy is especially indicated in behalf of nervous people of sedentary habits; also so-called bilious people, and those who suffer from chronic dyspepsia, from chronic constipation, and from chronic hypochondriacal melancholia; mental depression from overstudy, from overanxiety, and from overdrinking; loss of mental power from masturbation, and from excessive indulgence with those of the opposite sex. It produces favourable results in the cases of many people who suffer from hard work, personal neglect, unnaturally irascible tempers, drinking and debauchery, mental depression, and from pessimistic views of life. Its administration is efficacious in the relief of sleeplessness in such patients as we have just described, if they will simply reverse their methods of living, and correct their daily habits, and make them conform, to a reasonable extent, with the simple but positive requirements of nature.

OPIUM

General Action.—It produces a general depression, torpor and paralysis of functional activity; it befogs the mental faculties, impedes the action of the heart, and diminishes the secretions of the mucous membranes.

Brain and Spinal Cord.—Congestion of the brain; vertigo, as if intoxicated; pressive pains in the head and cold sweat upon the forehead; cold extremities, numbness and trembling of the limbs; spasms in the muscles of the back, causing the spine to curve like an arch.

Mind.—Dulness, stupidity, loss of consciousness; the patient acts as if in a drunken stupor; again, the patient becomes delirious, and has hallucinations of sight, and sees frightful visions; vivid imaginations; exaltations of mind; thinks herself away from home; apprehensive and frightened at seeing small animals; marked inability to tell the truth; Opium eaters are cunning and inveterate liars.

Sleep.—Deep, heavy sleep that is unrefreshing; sleeplessness from extreme sensitiveness of special senses; sleepless but stupid (also Gelsemium).

Accompaniments.—Chronic constipations from paralytic inactivity of the bowels; apoplectic conditions; spasmodic griping, pressive pains in abdomen; slow respiration; slow pulse with sharp pains through the chest.

Special Sphere of Action.—This drug is homeopathically applicable in the treatment of those who have long been dissipated; old people who are inclined to apoplexy or paralysis; melancholia, when the patients are at one time stupid and depressed, and again restless, anxious and troubled with vivid hallucinations of sight.

PHOSPHORIC ACID

General Action.—Acts upon the vegetative system, producing waste of tissue, and marked disturbance of the kidneys and male sexual organs. Under Phosphoric Acid the male sexual organs become relaxed, and unable to perform their natural functions.

Brain and Spinal Cord.—Sense of depression, with confusion and dulness of the brain; weakness in the back and limbs.

Mind.—Absolutely indifferent to surroundings; unable to think; disinclined to talk; loss of memory; questions are answered very slowly.

Sleep.—Drowsy and apathetic night and day, but sleep less after midnight.

Accompaniments.—Profuse urination; loss of appetite;

weakness of sexual organs; debilitating emissions; exhaustion after coition or masturbation.

Special Sphere of Action.—Dementia from masturbation, or from sexual excesses; palpitation of the heart in young people; melancholia from disappointment in love, from excessive menstruation, and from physical exhaustion due to overaction of the kidneys.

PHOSPHORUS

General Action.—It inflames and degenerates the mucous membranes of the entire alimentary tract; it produces an active parenchymatous degeneration of the liver; it destroys bone, especially the inferior maxilla and tibia; it causes fatty degeneration of all tissues of the body, leads to purpuric extravasations through disorganization of the blood; produces sanguineous infiltrations of lung tissue, and inflames the kidneys.

Brain and Spinal Cord.—Softening of the brain and spinal cord, with persistent headache; acute atrophy of the brain and the medulla oblongata; congestion of the brain, with throbbing of the temples; heat and burning in the brain and spine; weakness and heaviness in the limbs.

Mind.—Apathy, stupidity, indifference to everything; indisposition to mental or physical exertion (also Nux Vomica and Sulphur); ideas slow in evolution; inability to think; occasionally nervous, fearful and hysterical.

Sleep.—Sleepless before midnight; falls asleep, but awakens easily many times during the night.

Accompaniments.—Hoarseness; hollow, spasmodic cough; expectorations streaked with blood; short, labored respiration; great weakness, prostration and emaciation.

General Sphere of Action.—Insanity from masturbation or excessive sexual indulgence; insanity resulting from phthisis; cerebral softening; spinal softening; locomotor ataxia; paralysis following wasting diseases. It tends to delay the processes of cerebral degeneration, and hence it is of great value not only in relieving the sleeplessness of those suffering with organic brain disease, but it tends to ward off and hold in check approaching apoplexy and paralysis. It is sometimes combined with other drugs; and a useful constitutional remedy, and a nutrition-improving remedy is found in Calcarea Phosphorica. Also the brain fag of strong but overtaxed mental workers is relieved by the use of Phosphide of Zinc. But Phosphorus itself is a wonder-working brain remedy if judiciously applied. The sleeplessness of Phosphorus is characterized by short naps, and frequent waking during the night.

PLATINA

General Action.—Acts upon the nerve centers, producing depression of the sensorium and derangement of the entire nervous system.

Brain and Spinal Cord.—Sensation of numbness or coldness in the head; sensation in the temples, as if the head was tightly bound, or as if the various parts were closely screwed together; sensation of cold spots on the temples.

Mind.—Full of unnecessary pride; looks with contempt upon those around her; fancies herself great, and that her neighbors are small, insignificant and weaker than herself in both mind and body; at times depressed, inclined to weep, feels lonesome, but too proud to associate with her friends.

Sleep.—Indulges much in spasmodic yawnings; is very sleepy, but sleep is light and often broken.

Accompaniments.—Inflammation of the ovaries, with paroxysms of burning pain; sensitiveness of the female genital organs; voluptuous inclinations, with anxiety and palpitation of the heart.

Special Sphere of Action.—Mania with pride; melancholia complicated with hysteria; nymphomania due to inflammation of the ovaries. The drug is especially adapted to the treatment of hysterical females. It is often given for monomanias of pride and grandeur. These patients are haughty and dictatorial, overbearing and faultfinding; look down disdainfully on others.

PODOPHYLLUM

General Action.—Its chief action is upon the abdominal viscera, resulting in a profuse, forcibly ejected diarrhea, and a secondary torpor, and congestion of the liver. Reflexly, symptoms of cerebral irritation follow.

Brain and Spinal Cord.—Vertigo, with sensation of falling forward; headache; rolls the head and moans; pain between the shoulders, and along the spine in the morning.

Mind.—Depression of spirits; imagines that he is going to die; has a disgust for life on account of tormenting gastric difficulties.

Sleep.—Heavy sleep; vertigo on awakening; moaning in sleep (also Belladonna).

Accompaniments.—Diarrhea, with frequent, yellow, painless stools, stools with a meal-like sediment; sour smelling stools, with flatulence; bloody stools, with prolapsus ani; diarrhea worse in the morning. On the other hand, there may be constipation, with clay-colored or chalky stools (Mercury); general appearance of jaundice; dyspepsia; yellow coated tongue; alternation of diarrhea and constipation (also Nux Vomica).

Special Sphere of Action.—Hypochondriacal melancholia

PULSATILLA

General Action.—Pulsatilla, through the cerebro-spinal system, works its effects upon the mucous and serous membranes, upon the veins, upon the generative organs of both sexes, upon the ears and eyes. Among its general effects are increased catarrhal discharges from all mucous surfaces.

Brain and Spinal Cord.—The brain symptoms seem to rise by reflex action from diseased conditions of other organs of the body; there is headache, with suppression of the menses; headache from over-loaded stomach, especially after eating fat food; headache after catarrh of the nasal and bronchial air passages; stiffness and rheumatic pains in the nape of the neck; pain in the small of the back as from a sprain; hip joint painful as if dislocated; drawing, tensive pain in the thighs and legs.

Mind.—Constant inclination to weep; gentle, timid and yielding disposition; at the same time fretful, morose, and easily put out of sorts. Fretfulness and fearfulness are the chief characteristics of the Pulsatilla patient.

Sleep.—Sleeplessness from effects of late suppers, or from eating too much; sleepless the first half of the night; sleeps freely toward morning; screaming and whining in sleep on account of vivid or frightful dreams.

Special Sphere of Action.—Pulsatilla is a remedy of frequent service among insane women who suffer with disordered menstruation. Pulsatilla patients are of a mild, gentle, yielding disposition, disposed to cheerfulness, and yet manifesting a changeable and fickle disposition, often smiling in the midst of tears. When the menses are delayed or absent, Pulsatilla is of great service in establishing the flow, and among insane women this is frequently followed by improvement in the mental symptoms. Religious melancholia, especially in women who are weak in body, and anxious and apprehensive in mind. It is especially applicable to those states of hypochondriacal depression preceded or accompanied by profuse catarrhal discharges, and by inflammatory conditions of the genital organs in both sexes; acute glandular affections, particularly in the breasts and testicles; recent gastric disorders; inflammatory states of the eye and ear.

RHUS TOXICODENDRON

General Action.—Acts upon the cerebro-spinal system; upon the skin, the lymphatic glands, and the muscular tissues; it produces conditions simulating rheumatism, erysipelas, and typhus fever.

Brain and Spinal Cord.—Congestive headache, with burning in the ears and vertex; vesicular eruptions upon the scalp; fulness and heaviness, and sensation of weight in the forehead; rheumatic pains in the back and joints of the shoulder, arm and wrist; fulness and pain in the limbs on first moving in the morning; relieved by constant motion.

Mind.—Absence of mind; forgetful, difficulty in remembering the most recent events; apprehensiveness; anxiety, with restlessness; cannot stay in bed; delirium; thinks he is walking over large fields; suicidal and wants to drown herself; fears she is being poisoned.

Sleep.—Repeated yawning, without being sleepy; dreams of taking severe exercise, and awakens very much exhausted as a result of these dreams.

Accompaniments.—Diseases of a rheumatic nature; erysipelas, with mild delirium; eruptions upon the skin of a vesicular type; great debility, with restlessness; fever of a rheumatic type, with marked cerebral disturbance.

Special Sphere of Action.—Mental depression in rheumatic patients, with great physical res ssness; delirium accompanying diseases which result from exposure to storms.

SECALE CORNUTUM

General Action.—Acts upon the cerebro-spinal system, and upon the great sympathetic system; it affects the vasomotor nerves and causes contraction of the coats of the blood vessels. The contractions are followed by relaxations and by irregular dilations of the blood vessels. Secale also produces blood disorganization, and gangrene of the extremities.

Brain and Spinal Cord.—Congestion of tne brain, and vertigo; subsequently, it causes cerebral and spinal anemia; pain and confusion in the head; sensation as if the contents of the skull were being washed about; spinal paralysis with rapid emaciation; spasmodic jerkings of paralyzed limbs; painful contractions of flexor muscles; tingling in limbs; sensation as if ants were crawling over the skin.

Mind.—Apathetic, stupid, unable to think quickly; from a dull mental state the patient sometimes rises to a condition of mania with inclination to bite. Again, there is great depression of mind, with sadness and fear of death; yet with this fear of death there are, oftentimes, suicidal tendencies (also Arsenicum), especially by drowning.

Sleep.—Drowsiness; stupor, with frequent yawning; great inclination to sleep, but sleep is disturbed by frightful dreams.

Accompaniments.—Uterine hemorrhage, prostration of strength; tendency to emaciation; small, rapid, and sometimes fluttering pulse; anxious, labored inspiration, with constant tendency to sigh; cold extremities; cramps in limbs, and sometimes convulsions.

Special Sphere of Action.—This drug is particularly adapted to the relief of mental diseases occurring in weak and scrawny women, in feeble and aged persons, or in those who have become, by effects of disease, prematurely old. It is useful in mental depressions after hemorrhages and other exhausting bodily disorders.

SEPIA

General Action.—It acts apparently upon the great sympathetic system; it produces congestive effects upon the female sexual organs, and upon the liver. It also induces cerebral anemia.

Brain and Spinal Cord.—Boring headache accompanied by vertigo; shooting pains in the head; hemicrania; sensation as if the head would burst; aggravated by stooping, coughing, or motion; pain in small of the back, with much stiffness; pain relieved by walking (also Rhus Toxicodendron); heaviness and weakness of the limbs.

Mind.—Sensitive and sad; much inclined to weep (also Natrum Muriaticum and Pulsatilla); at times apathetic and indifferent; again fretful and easily offended; dread of being alone; apprehensive of the future, and has great fears concerning her health.

Sleep.—Sleepy during the daytime and early in the evening; awakens at three A.M., and cannot sleep again; (Nux Vomica patient wakens at three A.M., but after a time falls asleep, and sleeps till late in the morning); talks loudly in sleep; sleepless from rush of thoughts; awakens at night, with palpitation and anxiety about things happened years ago.

Accompaniments.—Yellow, waxy complexion, with general puffed appearance of the face; yellow spots on the skin; pains in the uterus, with a sensation as if the contents of the pelvis would protrude through the vulva. Dyspepsia, with an all-gone sensation in the pit of the stomach; excessive prostration after uterine disease.

Special Sphere of Action.—Sepia is a valuable remedy for mild cases of melancholia in chlorotic, puffy, and pot-bellied women, and for those who have suffered from miscarriages, from difficult labors, from profuse menses, and chronic leucorrhea. It is valuable for mental depression following the condition known as subinvolution of the uterus.

SILICEA

General Action.—It acts upon the sympathetic system, and produces marked effects upon the glandular structures, the bones, and the mucous surfaces. Silicea has a marked control over the suppurative process.

Brain and Spinal Cord.—Headache from congestion of the brain, with excessive sensitiveness of the nervous system; headache aggravated by noise, motion and stooping; headache produced by the excitement of the passions; the headache is severe, throbbing, shooting and burning in character; the Silicea headache is usually circumscribed, and may affect the occiput, the vertex, or the forehead; the Silicea headache is relieved by warmth, and by carefully binding up the head with a cloth (also Argentum Nitricum); the spine is sensitive to touch; there is formication of the limbs, and a feeling of weakness in walking, produced by spinal debility.

Mind.—Weak-minded; desponding; low-spirited; wishes to drown herself; compunctions of conscience about trifles; yielding disposition; faint-hearted; has no "sand".

Sleep.—Somnambulism; has anxious dreams of murder; has lascivious dreams; jerkings of the limbs during sleep.

Accompaniments.—Abdomen hard and tense; constipation; attempts at stool are but partially successful; swollen and hardened glands; great debility; ulcers, with stinging burning, pains; small wounds heal with great difficulty.

Special Sphere of Action.—It is indicated in profound melancholia with symptoms like the foregoing; in melancholia accompanied by boils, carbuncles, abscesses, ulcers, or swollen glands. When we wish to remove or relieve deep-seated and long-lasting effects of defective assimilation, we think of Silicea. It corresponds well with what the older writers called the "scrofulous diathesis", attended by suppurative processes affecting either the glands or the osseous system. It is also a safe and useful remedy in epilepsy, where the causes arise from maldevelopment, and where aggravations occur either weekly or monthly.

SPONGIA

General Action.—It produces enlargements and indurations of the ductless glands, especially the thyroid, with irritation of the trachea and larynx.

Brain and Spinal Cord.—Congestion of the brain; dull headache on the right side; sharp stitches in the temples; painful stiffness in the muscles of the neck and back; twitchings in the muscles of the limbs; exhaustion and heaviness of the muscles of the limbs; exhaustion and heaviness of the body after the slightest exertion.

Mind.—Irresistible desire to sing; the Spongia patient is jolly like Hyoscyamus, but the gaiety of spirits is longer continued and less variable than in Hyoscyamus.

Sleep.—Sleepy during the day; sleep interrupted by dreams at night.

Accompaniments.—Great difficulty in breathing; hoarse,

hollow cough; the patient is wheezing and asthmatic, and yet constantly inclined to sing.

Special Sphere of Action.—Mania, with gaiety of spirits; women and children who are lighthearted and hopeful, but who have strong tendencies to phthisis.

STRAMONIUM

General Action.—Acts upon the sensorium, stimulating it to undue activity, and inducing hallucinations of sight and hearing of the most vivid character; it also produces suppression of urine; great sexual excitement; tendency to convulsions; fiery eruptions of the skin, dryness of the throat, with fear of water.

Brain and Spinal Cord.—Violent congestion of the brain; excessive heat in the head; pulsations in the forehead, but less violent than those induced by Belladonna; twitchings of the hands and feet, and trembling of the limbs; cataleptic states.

Mind.—Extraordinary mental excitement; sudden and kaleidoscopic changes in the mental state; at times full of horrible fears; at times merry, and enjoying himself by singing and dancing; at times proud, haughty, and intolerant of those around him; at times full of rage, trying to strike with great vigor those within his reach; and again, dulness of the senses, with stupid indifference to every thing about him. Fear and hope, jollity and rage, frenzy and apathy follow each other in rapid succession under Stramonium; the passions and the mental manifestations become strangely jumbled in their exhibition under the influence of this stimulating drug. The Stramonium patient desires light and company, and at the same time is often terrified by bright objects, and seeks to fight those whom he constantly wishes to have in his presence. He has hallucinations of sight during which horrible images are conjured up, and horrible animals are seen jumping out of the ground and running at their affrighted victim.

Sleep.—Deep, heavy sleep, with snoring or stertorous breathing; the heavy sleep is short, and the patient is often roused, apparently by seeing horrible objects in his dreams; twitching and cramping during sleep.

Accompaniments.—Suppression of urine; convulsions from the sight of bright objects; trembling of the whole body as if from fright; difficulty of deglutition; spasms are often excited when water is placed at the lips of the Stramonium patient; under Stramonium, the sexual desires of both sexes are greatly increased.

Special Sphere of Action.—Chorea, epilepsy, hydrophobia, hysteria, delirium tremens, and, most of all, acute mania when the patient rises to a condition of mental frenzy, far surpassing the exaltation of the Hyoscyamus case, but when the actual inflammatory condition of the cerebrum is of a milder degree than that found under Belladonna. This remedy will be found of service when the patient is greatly agitated and extremely fearful of everything that he hears or sees. He has the horrors, so to speak, and is in constant dread of being attacked by all kinds of terrible animals. One patient who at times imagines that snakes are pursuing her, has frequently been quieted, and this symptom dispelled by a few doses of Stramonium. The nurse in charge has noticed this effect, and when the vision of snakes appears to this patient, she sends to the attending physician, and asks for some of the "snake medicine" for the patient. Stramonium is a remedy adapted to the relief of maniacal attacks which sometimes appear in paretics before or after epileptiform seizures.

STAPHISAGRIA

General Action.—It produces a chronic irritation and hyper-excitability of the male genital organs, particularly of the prostatic urethra and the adjacent seminal ducts; and secondarily develops all the physical and mental symptoms of spermatorrhea.

Brain and Spinal Cord.—Stupefying headache, or as if a round ball were in the forehead, which persists even when shaking the head.

Mind.—Very peevish; easily offended; becomes indignant; thinks the least thing done is a premeditated insult; hypochondriacal or apathetic mood; prefers solitude, and is shy of the opposite sex; obtuseness of mind; thoughts vanish while speaking or thinking.

Sleep.—Uneasy sleep, with anxious dreams, or dreams of the previous day's works. Amorous dreams, with seminal emissions.

Accompaniments.—Weak, pale and sallow, with dark rings beneath the eyes, from masturbation or excessive sexual intercourse. Great lassitude and indolence; eczematous eruptions; pains in the long bones; excoriating coryza, and relaxation of the alimentary canal, with desire for spices, wine or other stimulants.

Special Sphere of Action.—It finds its principal employment in removing the results of excessive masturbation in either sex. These cases are weak, fretful, lacking in self-control, unable to concentrate the mind; their nervous systems are exhausted, and their own ailments are the constant subject of their contemplation, and should, in their opinion, be a topic of unfailing interest to every one else.

SULPHUR

General Action.—It acts upon the ganglionic nervous system, and it works its effects most profoundly throughout the entire vegetative sphere. Every organ in the body is affected by the administration of Sulphur; but we look for its most prominent results in the skin, the mucous membranes, the lymphatic glands, and the venous circulation.

Brain and Spinal Cord.—Sulphur produces a rush of blood to the head; a pressive frontal headache, worse in the morning; headache in the vertex as from a weight; a headache with vertigo while walking or stooping; a headache, with great confusion in the head, and a sensation as if a band was bound around the forehead (also Cocculus and Mercurius); there is stiffness in the neck and back; bruised pain in the small of the back and the coccyx; tearing, drawing, rheumatic pains in the shoulders, arms and legs; burning in the soles of the feet.

Mind.—Intense anxiety and apprehension, especially in the evening (also Calcarea Carbonica); indulgences in philosophical speculations are followed by abnormal mental exhaustion, and an inability to hold his mind to work upon any subject; at times fretful and ill-humored; at times indolent and indisposed to exercise; at times sad, melancholy, inclined to weep, and despair of salvation.

Sleep.—Often wakeful during the entire night; when the patient does sleep he awakens frequently (also Phosphorus); anxious and vivid dreams accompanied by starting during sleep, especially soon after falling asleep; insufficient sleep at night, and irresistible drowsiness during the day.

Accompaniments.—Great sensitiveness of the scalp and skin generally; sensitiveness of the eyes to light; sensitiveness of the ears to loud noises; toothache, with great sensitiveness to cold water and cold air; distention of the abdomen from incarcerated flatulence, and great sensitiveness of the abdomen to touch; hoarseness; dry cough in the evening or on waking; pains and sensitiveness in the joints. The Sulphur patient is sensitive in all his organs, and is opposed to all external impressions. He dreads exercise or contact with others; he dreads fresh air; he dreads to take a bath, on account of being so intensely sensitive.

Special Sphere of Action.—Sulphur is particularly adapted to lean, sensitive and phthisical persons who are inclined to religious melancholy; such patients become depressed and discouraged because their minds are constantly disturbed by every impression or experience in life. We are obliged to prescribe Sulphur for the insane more on account of the external symptoms than because of any special mental characteristics. As a characteristic of the Sulphur patient, it has been said that he uses his sleeves both for "handkerchief and looking-glass". He is dirty, and looks dirty; has an aversion to water, and to washing; the skin is harsh and unclean; the habits are untidy. Mentally, he is irritable and a chronic grumbler. Sulphur is frequently useful in the treatment of patients with chronic mania who attach great value to trifling objects, who dress themselves up in rags, wear paper crowns, and imagine that they are kings and queens. The Sulphur patient is selfish, and is anxious about his own salvation, but indifferent to that of others. In cases of this sort, Sulphur is useful as a constitutional remedy, and it prepares the system for the beneficial effects of other remedies. When mental symptoms are not well pronounced in a case of insanity, a few doses of Sulphur will often lead the patient to disclose characteristic conditions of the mind, and insane delusions which have heretofore been concealed.

THUJA

General Action.—It produces a tendency to acrid secretions, especially about the anus and genital organs; constitutionally, it produces partial disorganization of the blood, and a tendency to wasting of tissue.

Brain and Spinal Cord.—Dull confusion in the head; vertigo as soon as the eyes are closed, or upon suddenly turning the head. (Lachesis has vertigo from looking steadily at one object). Headache as if a nail were driven into the head (also Ignatia).

Mind.—Disinclined to be touched or even approached; thinks he is made of brittle material and may break; thinks his limbs are separated (also Baptisia); or that a living animal inhabits his abdomen, which he feels moving there. Either hurried in manner and ill-humored, or is unable to recall needed words, and is slow in speech and thought.

Sleep.—Falls asleep late owing to persistent restlessness; lascivious dreams without emission of semen, wakes unrefreshed.

Accompaniments.—Warty growth upon the skin or mucous membranes, seedy or cauliflower-like in structure. Sight blurred; sees apparitions upon closing the eyes; greenish yellow gonorrhea; neuralgia, beginning over the eye, and seeming to extend backward over the head. (Gelsemium and Spigelia extend forward).

Special Sphere of Action.—It is called for in states of mental depression and apathy, with desire to be left alone, when this frame of mind follows direct and personal knowledge that the way of the transgressor is hard. Thuja corrects the physical susceptibility which adds to the severity of non-syphilitic venereal diseases, and removes the lowness of spirits, self-depreciation and loathing of life which is often found with severe disease of the sexual organs. In ordinary hypochondriacal melancholia the delusion that a living creature is in the abdomen, or that his members are changed in structure, will not infrequently guide to its successful application.

VERATRUM ALBUM

General Action.—This drug acts upon the cerebro-spinal system, at times to the extent of producing convulsions; it disorganizes the blood, and impairs the circulation; it produces collapse, vomiting, purging, spasmodic, and clammy perspiration.

Brain and Spinal Cord.—Congestion of the brain when stooping; headache as if the head would burst; dull pressure in the vertex; coldness as if ice were on the vertex; paralytic weakness of the limbs; limbs feel as if asleep; hands and feet feel bruised and icy cold; cramps in the calves of the legs.

Mind.—Anxiety and apprehension; a tendency to weep, and howl, and scream over some dreaded misfortune; tendency to tear and cut clothing; when the rage of mania subsides, there is a tendency to converse about religious matters; the religious natures of the Veratrum patients become chameleonhued in their manifestations; they pray and curse in alternation for many hours in succession; finally these patients despair of salvation, and of their position in society. When disengaged from religious contemplation, the Veratrum patients are inclined to gossip, to find fault with others, to scold their friends, and to call their neighbors hard names. The Veratrum patient sometimes fancies herself pregnant, even when eighty or ninety years of age.

Sleep.—At times very sleepy and drowsy; at times exalted and sleepless for days and nights in succession, sleeplessness from undue mental activity, preceding a state of physical collapse.

Accompaniments.—Pale, sunken face, with blue nose

and cold perspiration on the forehead; violent vomiting, first of food, and then of green, slimy, viscid liquid; profuse, painful and violent diarrhea; discharges sudden and involuntary, with cramping pains in the bowels, and in the calves of the legs; great difficulty in respiration; palpitation of the heart, with anxiety; sudden failure of the strength; extreme prostration, with coldness and a tendency to cramps.

Special Sphere of Action.—Acute mania with rapid exhaustion; acute dementia with prostration and coldness of the extremities; acute melancholia with intense anxiety and despair of salvation, particularly in women whose menses have been suppressed, or in women who fancy themselves pregnant.

VERATRUM VIRIDE

General Action.—Acts upon the cerebro-spinal system, and especially upon the pneumogastric nerve, disturbing the circulatory apparatus, and causing congestion and inflammation of the brain and other organs; it produces intense prostration and tendency to spasms; it causes a strong beating of the heart, and a quick pulse, but a slow respiration.

Brain and Spinal Cord.—Headache proceeding from the nape of the neck; active congestion of the brain, followed by vomiting; cutting pains in the neck and shoulders; cramps in the legs and hands; shocks like electricity pass rapidly through the limbs; convulsive twitchings of all the muscles of the extremities.

Mind.—Intensely quarrelsome and delirious; from a condition of excitability and quarrelsomeness the patient passes into a state in which she is sullen, suspicious, and distrustful of those around her; the Veratrum Viride patient has in mind a constant fear that she will be insane (also Sepia, Calcarea Carbonica and Lilium Tigrinum); also thinks she will be poisoned.

Sleep.—Restless each night, but generally secures some sleep; is disturbed by frightful dreams of being on the water; and of being drowned.

Accompaniments.—Convulsions before, during and after labor; intense nausea and vomiting; cutting neuralgic pains in the abdomen; profuse urine, which is pale; active congestion of the chief organs of the body; slow, weak pulse, or palpitation, with fluttering sensation in region of the heart, with quick pulse.

Special Sphere of Action.—Puerperal mania; general paresis; particularly after convulsions; epileptic mania, with frequent convulsive attacks; hysterical mania; melancholia, with a tendency to chorea; melancholia or mania following cerebro-spinal fever.

ZINCUM METALLICUM

General Action.—Its general action resembles that of lead in the physical weakness produced through nerve exhaustion and anemia. The cerebro-spinal system is most affected.

Brain and Spinal Cord.—Sharp, lancinating headaches low in the occiput, or in the root of the nose. Burning pain along the whole course of the spinal cord; a sense of formication in the limbs; cannot hold the feet still; the muscles jerk voluntarily; the hands tremble; sharp pains are experienced along the course of the peripheral nerves.

Mind.—Sad, morose and dejected, with thoughts of death, which he considers indifferently and without fear; or, fretful and irritable, with great aversion to noise; starts at every unexpected sound. Again, there may be difficulty in comprehending, which leads the patient to repeat all questions before endeavoring to answer.

Sleep.—Sleeps poorly; dreams of filth, of being pursued, or of terrifying experiences; wakes in a fright.

Accompaniments.—Nausea and vomiting as soon as food touches the stomach; hydræmia, venous congestions, and a tendency to varicose veins in the extremities; dryness and thickening of the skin.

Special Sphere of Action.—When prolonged mental overwork and close confinement have produced a state of forgetfulness, mental weakness, inability to apply the mind, broken and unrefreshing sleep, Zincum becomes a most valuable remedy, aided by rest, and change of scene. Many cases of melancholia present mental exhaustion as their immediate cause, and are helped by its administration; and it is used when defective reaction and lack of trophic power retard recovery.

INDEX

OF REMEDIES WITH THEIR PRINCIPAL SYMPTOMS

Remedy	Page
ACONITE	237-9
Mania, Melancholia	
AGARICUS MUSCARIUS	239-40
ALUMINA	240-1
ANACARDIUM	241-2
Dementia, Mental weakness	
ANTIMONIUM CRUDUM	242-3
ANTIMONIUM TARTARICUM	243-4
APIS MELLIFICA	244-5
Dementia	
ARGENTUM NITRICUM	245-6
ARNICA	246-7
ARSENICUM	247-9
Mania, Melancholia, Neuralgia, Sleeplessness	
AURUM METALLICUM	249-50
Melancholia	
BAPTISIA	250-1
Mania	
BELLADONNA	251-2
Mania, Sleeplessness	
BRYONIA	252-3
Peevishness	
CACTUS GRANDIFLORUS	254
Melancholia	
CALCAREA CARBONICUM	254-6
Dementia	
CALCAREA PHOSPHORICUM	256
CAMPHOR	256-7
CANNABIS INDICA	257-8
CANTHARIS	258-60
Mania	
CAUSTICUM	260-1
CHAMOMILLA	261-2
Peevishness, Sleeplessness	
CHINA	262-3
CICUTA VIROSA	263-4
CIMICIFUGA	264-5
Melancholia, Sleeplessness	
COCCULUS	265-6
COFFEA CRUDA	266-7
COLCHICUM	267
COLOCYNTH	268
CONIUM MACULATUM	268-9
CUPRUM METALLICUM	269-70
DIGITALIS	270-1
Melancholia	
FERRUM METALLICUM	271-2
GELSEMIUM	272-3
Melancholia, Sleeplessness	
GLONOIN	273-4
HELLEBORUS NIGER	274
HEPAR SULPHUR	275
HYOSCYAMUS	275-7
Mania, Sleeplessness	
HYPERICUM	277
IGNATIA	278-9
Melancholia	
IODINE	279-80
LACHESIS	280-2
Mania	

INDEX

	Page		Page
Lilium Tigrinum	282-3	Rhus Toxicodendron	295-6
Melancholia		Secale Cornutum	296-7
Lycopodium	283-4	Sepia	297-8
Mercurius	284-5	Melancholia	
Natrum Muriaticum	286-7	Silicea	298-9
Melancholia		Epilepsy	
Nitric Acid	287	Spongia	299-300
Nux Vomica	288-9	Stramonium	300-1
Sleeplessness, Subacute mania		Mania, Sleeplessness	
Opium	289-90	Staphisagria	302
Melancholia, Mental weakness		Sulphur	302-3
		Mania	
Phosphoric Acid	290-1	Thuja	304-6
Mental weakness, Dementia		Veratrum Album	306-7
Phosphorus	291-2	History, Mania, Melancholia, Sleeplessness	
Platina	292-3		
Podophyllum	293-4	Veratrum Viride	307-8
Pulsatilla	294-5	Mania	
Melancholia		Zincum Metallicum	308-9